Underground Clinical Vignettes

Microbiology II: Bacteriology

FIFTH EDITION

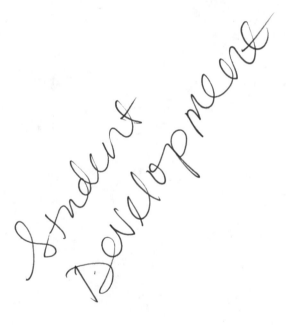

Underground
Clinical Vignettes
Microbiology II: Bacteriology

FIFTH EDITION

Todd A. Swanson, M.D., Ph.D.
Resident in Radiation Oncology
William Beaumont Hospital
Royal Oak, Michigan

Sandra I. Kim, M.D., Ph.D.
Resident in Internal Medicine
Beth Israel Deaconess Medical Center
Harvard Medical School
Boston, Massachusetts

Olga E. Flomin, M.D.
Resident in Obstetrics and Gynecology
William Beaumont Hospital
Royal Oak, Michigan

Wolters Kluwer | Lippincott Williams & Wilkins
Health
Philadelphia · Baltimore · New York · London
Buenos Aires · Hong Kong · Sydney · Tokyo

Acquisitions Editor: Nancy Anastasi Duffy
Developmental Editor: Kathleen H. Scogna
Managing Editor: Nancy Hoffmann
Marketing Manager: Jennifer Kuklinski
Associate Production Manager: Kevin P. Johnson
Creative Director: Doug Smock
Compositor: International Typesetting and Composition
Printer: R.R. Donnelley & Son's—Crawfordsville

Printed in the United States of America

First Edition, 2001 Blackwell Publishing Inc.
Second Edition, 2003 Blackwell Publishing Inc.
Third Edition, 2005 Blackwell Publishing Inc.
Fourth Edition, 2005 Blackwell Publishing Inc.

Library of Congress Cataloging-in-Publication Data

Swanson, Todd A.
  Microbiology / Todd Swanson, Sandra Kim, Olga E. Flomin.—5th ed.
    p. ; cm.—(Underground clinical vignettes)
  Rev. ed. of: Microbiology / Vikas Bhushan . . . [et al.]. 4th ed. c2005.
  Includes bibliographical references and index.
  ISBN-13: 978-0-7817-6471-1 (alk. paper)
  ISBN-10: 0-7817-6471-8 (alk. paper)
  1. Medical microbiology—Case studies. 2. Physicians—Licenses—United States—Examinations—Study guides. I. Kim, Sandra. II. Flomin, Olga E. III. Microbiology.
IV Title. V. Series.
  [DNLM: 1. Microbiology—Case Reports. 2. Microbiology—Problems and Exercises.
QW 18.2 S972m 2007]
  QR46.B465 2007
  616.9'041—dc22

2007003561

06 07 08 09 10
1 2 3 4 5 6 7 8 9 10

dedications

For Natan and Marina,
for whose encouragement and assistance we are eternally grateful.

preface

First published in 1999, the *Underground Clinical Vignettes* (UCV) series has provided thousands of students with a highly effective review tool as they prepare for medical exams, particularly the USMLE Step 1 and 2 exams. Designed as a quick study guide, each UCV book contains patient-centered clinical cases that highlight a range of medical diagnoses.

With this new edition of UCV, we have incorporated feedback from medical students across the country to provide updated cases with expanded treatment and discussion sections. A new two-page format enables readers to formulate an initial diagnosis prior to reading the answer, while the added differential diagnosis section encourages critical thinking about comparable cases. The inclusion of relevant MRI images, x-rays, and photographs allows students to more readily visualize the physical presentation of each case. Breakout boxes, tables, and algorithms have been added, along with all new Board format QAs, making this edition of UCV an ideal source of information for exam review, classroom discussion, or clinical rotations.

The clinical vignettes in this series are designed to give added emphasis to pathogenesis, epidemiology, management, and complications. Although each case tends to present all the signs, symptoms, and diagnostic findings for a particular illness, patients generally will not present with such a "complete" picture either clinically or on a medical examination. Cases are not meant to simulate a potential real patient or an exam vignette.

Access to LWW's online companion site, ThePoint, will be offered as a premium with the purchase of the Underground Clinical Vignettes Step 1 bundle. Benefits include an online test link and additional new Board format questions covering all UCV subject areas.

We hope you will find the Underground Clinical Vignettes series informative and useful. We welcome any feedback, suggestions, or corrections you have about this series. Please contact us at LWW.com/medstudent.

contributors

Series Editors

Todd A. Swanson, M.D., Ph.D.
Resident in Radiation Oncology
William Beaumont Hospital
Royal Oak, Michigan

Sandra I. Kim, M.D., Ph.D.
Resident in Internal Medicine
Beth Israel Deaconess Medical Center
Harvard Medical School
Boston, Massachusetts

Series Contributors

Olga E. Flomin, M.D.
Resident in Obstetrics and Gynecology
William Beaumont Hospital
Royal Oak, Michigan

Medina C. Kushen, M.D.
Resident in Neurosurgery
University of Chicago Hospitals
Chicago, Illinois

Marc J. Glucksman, Ph.D.
Professor of Biochemistry and Molecular Biology
Director, Midwest Proteome Center and
Co-Director, Rosalind Franklin Structural Biology Laboratories
Rosalind Franklin University of Medicine and Science
The Chicago Medical School
North Chicago, Illinois

acknowledgments

Thanks to Dr. Alvaro Martinez, Dr. Larry Kestin, and the entire radiation oncology program at William Beaumont Hospital for allowing the flexibility to work on this project during an already vigorous residency training program.

—Todd A. Swanson

Thanks to Todd for his work on this series.

—Sandra I. Kim

abbreviations

ABGs	arterial blood gases	BPH	benign prostatic hypertrophy
ABPA	allergic bronchopulmonary aspergillosis	BUN	blood urea nitrogen
		CABG	coronary artery bypass grafting
ACA	anticardiolipin antibody	CAD	coronary artery disease
ACE	angiotensin-converting enzyme	CaEDTA	calcium edetate
ACL	anterior cruciate ligament	CALLA	common acute lymphoblastic leukemia antigen
ACTH	adrenocorticotropic hormone		
AD	adjustment disorder	cAMP	cyclic adenosine monophosphate
ADA	adenosine deaminase		
ADD	attention deficit disorder	C-ANCA	cytoplasmic antineutrophil cytoplasmic antibody
ADH	antidiuretic hormone		
ADHD	attention deficit hyperactivity disorder	CBC	complete blood count
		CBD	common bile duct
ADP	adenosine diphosphate	CCU	cardiac care unit
AFO	ankle-foot orthosis	CD	cluster of differentiation
AFP	α-fetoprotein	2-CdA	2-chlorodeoxyadenosine
AIDS	acquired immunodeficiency syndrome	CEA	carcinoembryonic antigen
		CFTR	cystic fibrosis transmembrane conductance regulator
ALL	acute lymphocytic leukemia		
ALS	amyotrophic lateral sclerosis	cGMP	cyclic guanosine monophosphate
ALT	alanine aminotransferase		
AML	acute myelogenous leukemia	CHF	congestive heart failure
ANA	antinuclear antibody	CK	creatine kinase
Angio	angiography	CK-MB	creatine kinase, MB fraction
AP	anteroposterior	CLL	chronic lymphocytic leukemia
APKD	adult polycystic kidney disease	CML	chronic myelogenous leukemia
aPTT	activated partial thromboplastin time	CMV	cytomegalovirus
		CN	cranial nerve
ARDS	adult respiratory distress syndrome	CNS	central nervous system
		COPD	chronic obstructive pulmonary disease
5-ASA	5-aminosalicylic acid		
ASCA	antibodies to *Saccharomyces cerevisiae*	COX	cyclooxygenase
		CP	cerebellopontine
ASO	antistreptolysin O	CPAP	continuous positive airway pressure
AST	aspartate aminotransferase		
ATLL	adult T-cell leukemia/lymphoma	CPK	creatine phosphokinase
ATPase	adenosine triphosphatase	CPPD	calcium pyrophosphate dihydrate
AV	arteriovenous, atrioventricular		
AZT	azidothymidine (zidovudine)	CPR	cardiopulmonary resuscitation
BAL	British antilewisite (dimercaprol)	CREST	calcinosis, Raynaud phenomenon, esophageal involvement, sclerodactyly, telangiectasia (syndrome)
BCG	bacille Calmette-Guérin		
BE	barium enema		
b.i.d.	twice a day		
BP	blood pressure	CRP	C-reactive protein

CSF	cerebrospinal fluid	ENT	ears, nose, and throat
CSOM	chronic suppurative otitis media	EPVE	early prosthetic valve endocarditis
CT	cardiac transplant, computed tomography	ER	emergency room
		ERCP	endoscopic retrograde cholangiopancreatography
CVA	cerebrovascular accident		
CXR	chest x-ray	ERT	estrogen replacement therapy
d4T	didehydrodeoxythymidine (stavudine)	ESR	erythrocyte sedimentation rate
		ETEC	enterotoxigenic *E. coli*
DCS	decompression sickness	EtOH	ethanol
DDH	developmental dysplasia of the hip	FAP	familial adenomatous polyposis
		FEV_1	forced expiratory volume in 1 second
ddI	dideoxyinosine (didanosine)		
DES	diethylstilbestrol	FH	familial hypercholesterolemia
DEXA	dual-energy x-ray absorptiometry	FNA	fine-needle aspiration
DHEAS	dehydroepiandrosterone sulfate	FSH	follicle-stimulating hormone
DIC	disseminated intravascular coagulation	FTA-ABS	fluorescent treponemal antibody absorption test
DIF	direct immunofluorescence	FVC	forced vital capacity
DIP	distal interphalangeal (joint)	G6PD	glucose-6-phosphate dehydrogenase
DKA	diabetic ketoacidosis		
DL_{CO}	diffusing capacity of carbon monoxide	GABA	gamma-aminobutyric acid
		GERD	gastroesophageal reflux disease
DMSA	2,3-dimercaptosuccinic acid	GFR	glomerular filtration rate
DNA	deoxyribonucleic acid	GGT	gamma-glutamyltransferase
DNase	deoxyribonuclease	GH	growth hormone
2,3-DPG	2,3-diphosphoglycerate	GI	gastrointestinal
dsDNA	double-stranded DNA	GnRH	gonadotropin-releasing hormone
DSM	Diagnostic and Statistical Manual	GU	genitourinary
		GVHD	graft-versus-host disease
dsRNA	double-stranded RNA	HAART	highly active antiretroviral therapy
DTP	diphtheria, tetanus, pertussis (vaccine)	HAV	hepatitis A virus
		Hb	hemoglobin
DTPA	diethylenetriamine-penta-acetic acid	HbA-1C	hemoglobin A-1C
		HBsAg	hepatitis B surface antigen
DTs	delirium tremens	HBV	hepatitis B virus
DVT	deep venous thrombosis	hCG	human chorionic gonadotropin
EBV	Epstein-Barr virus	HCO_3	bicarbonate
ECG	electrocardiography	Hct	hematocrit
Echo	echocardiography	HCV	hepatitis C virus
ECM	erythema chronicum migrans	HDL	high-density lipoprotein
ECT	electroconvulsive therapy	HDL-C	high-density lipoprotein-cholesterol
EEG	electroencephalography		
EF	ejection fraction, elongation factor	HEENT	head, eyes, ears, nose, and throat (exam)
EGD	esophagogastroduodenoscopy		
EHEC	enterohemorrhagic *E. coli*	HELLP	hemolysis, elevated LFTs, low platelets (syndrome)
EIA	enzyme immunoassay		
ELISA	enzyme-linked immunosorbent assay	HFMD	hand, foot, and mouth disease
		HGPRT	hypoxanthine-guanine phosphoribosyltransferase
EM	electron microscopy		
EMG	electromyography	5-HIAA	5-hydroxyindoleacetic acid

HIDA	hepato-iminodiacetic acid (scan)
HIV	human immunodeficiency virus
HLA	human leukocyte antigen
HMG-CoA	hydroxymethylglutaryl-coenzyme A
HMP	hexose monophosphate
HPI	history of present illness
HPV	human papillomavirus
HR	heart rate
HRIG	human rabies immune globulin
HRS	hepatorenal syndrome
HRT	hormone replacement therapy
HSG	hysterosalpingography
HSV	herpes simplex virus
HTLV	human T-cell leukemia virus
HUS	hemolytic uremic syndrome
HVA	homovanillic acid
ICP	intracranial pressure
ICU	intensive care unit
ID/CC	identification and chief complaint
IDDM	insulin-dependent diabetes mellitus
IFA	immunofluorescent antibody
Ig	immunoglobulin
IGF	insulin-like growth factor
IHSS	idiopathic hypertrophic subaortic stenosis
IM	intramuscular
IMA	inferior mesenteric artery
INH	isoniazid
INR	International Normalized Ratio
IP$_3$	inositol 1,4,5-triphosphate
IPF	idiopathic pulmonary fibrosis
ITP	idiopathic thrombocytopenic purpura
IUD	intrauterine device
IV	intravenous
IVC	inferior vena cava
IVIG	intravenous immunoglobulin
IVP	intravenous pyelography
JRA	juvenile rheumatoid arthritis
JVP	jugular venous pressure
KOH	potassium hydroxide
KUB	kidney, ureter, bladder
LCM	lymphocytic choriomeningitis
LDH	lactate dehydrogenase
LDL	low-density lipoprotein
LE	lupus erythematosus (cell)
LES	lower esophageal sphincter
LFTs	liver function tests

LH	luteinizing hormone
LMN	lower motor neuron
LP	lumbar puncture
LPVE	late prosthetic valve endocarditis
L/S	lecithin-sphingomyelin (ratio)
LSD	lysergic acid diethylamide
LT	labile toxin
LV	left ventricular
LVH	left ventricular hypertrophy
Lytes	electrolytes
Mammo	mammography
MAO	monoamine oxidase (inhibitor)
MCP	metacarpophalangeal (joint)
MCTD	mixed connective tissue disorder
MCV	mean corpuscular volume
MEN	multiple endocrine neoplasia
MI	myocardial infarction
MIBG	meta-iodobenzylguanidine (radioisotope)
MMR	measles, mumps, rubella (vaccine)
MPGN	membranoproliferative glomerulonephritis
MPS	mucopolysaccharide
MPTP	1-methyl-4-phenyl-tetrahydropy-ridine
MR	magnetic resonance (imaging)
mRNA	messenger ribonucleic acid
MRSA	methicillin-resistant *S. aureus*
MTP	metatarsophalangeal (joint)
NAD	nicotinamide adenine dinucleotide
NADP	nicotinamide adenine dinucleotide phosphate
NADPH	reduced nicotinamide adenine dinucleotide phosphate
NF	neurofibromatosis
NIDDM	non-insulin-dependent diabetes mellitus
NNRTI	non-nucleoside reverse tran-scriptase inhibitor
NO	nitric oxide
NPO	nil per os (nothing by mouth)
NSAID	nonsteroidal anti-inflammatory drug
Nuc	nuclear medicine
NYHA	New York Heart Association
OB	obstetric
OCD	obsessive-compulsive disorder
OCPs	oral contraceptive pills

OR	operating room	PTH	parathyroid hormone
PA	posteroanterior	PTSD	post-traumatic stress disorder
PABA	para-aminobenzoic acid	PTT	partial thromboplastin time
PAN	polyarteritis nodosa	PUVA	psoralen ultraviolet A
P-ANCA	perinuclear antineutrophil cyto-plasmic antibody	PVC	premature ventricular contraction
Pao_2	partial pressure of oxygen in arterial blood	q.i.d.	four times a day
		RA	rheumatoid arthritis
		RAIU	radioactive iodine uptake
PAS	periodic acid Schiff	RAST	radioallergosorbent test
PAT	paroxysmal atrial tachycardia	RBC	red blood cell
PBS	peripheral blood smear	REM	rapid eye movement
Pco_2	partial pressure of carbon dioxide	RES	reticuloendothelial system
PCOM	posterior communicating (artery)	RFFIT	rapid fluorescent focus inhibition test
PCOS	polycystic ovarian syndrome	RFTs	renal function tests
PCP	phencyclidine	RHD	rheumatic heart disease
PCR	polymerase chain reaction	RNA	ribonucleic acid
PCT	porphyria cutanea tarda	RNP	ribonucleoprotein
PCTA	percutaneous coronary translu-minal angioplasty	RPR	rapid plasma reagin
		RR	respiratory rate
PCV	polycythemia vera	RSV	respiratory syncytial virus
PDA	patent ductus arteriosus	RUQ	right upper quadrant
PDGF	platelet-derived growth factor	RV	residual volume
PE	physical exam	Sao_2	oxygen saturation in arterial blood
PEFR	peak expiratory flow rate		
PEG	polyethylene glycol	SBFT	small bowel follow-through
PEPCK	phosphoenolpyruvate carboxykinase	SCC	squamous cell carcinoma
		SCID	severe combined immunodeficiency
PET	positron emission tomography		
PFTs	pulmonary function tests	SERM	selective estrogen receptor modulator
PID	pelvic inflammatory disease		
PIP	proximal interphalangeal (joint)	SGOT	serum glutamic-oxaloacetic transaminase
PKU	phenylketonuria		
PMDD	premenstrual dysphoric disorder	SIADH	syndrome of inappropriate antidiuretic hormone
PML	progressive multifocal leukoen-cephalopathy		
		SIDS	sudden infant death syndrome
PMN	polymorphonuclear (leukocyte)	SLE	systemic lupus erythematosus
PNET	primitive neuroectodermal tumor	SMA	superior mesenteric artery
PNH	paroxysmal nocturnal hemoglobinuria	SSPE	subacute sclerosing panencephalitis
Po_2	partial pressure of oxygen	SSRI	selective serotonin reuptake inhibitor
PPD	purified protein derivative (of tuberculosis)		
		ST	stable toxin
PPH	primary postpartum hemorrhage	STD	sexually transmitted disease
PRA	panel reactive antibody	T2W	T2-weighted (MRI)
PROM	premature rupture of membranes	T_3	triiodothyronine
		T_4	thyroxine
PSA	prostate-specific antigen	TAH-BSO	total abdominal hysterectomy–bilateral salpingo-oophorectomy
PSS	progressive systemic sclerosis		
PT	prothrombin time	TB	tuberculosis

TCA	tricyclic antidepressant
TCC	transitional cell carcinoma
TDT	terminal deoxytransferase
TFTs	thyroid function tests
TGF	transforming growth factor
THC	tetrahydrocannabinol
TIA	transient ischemic attack
t.i.d.	three times a day
TIPS	transjugular intrahepatic portosystemic shunt
TLC	total lung capacity
TMP-SMX	trimethoprim-sulfamethoxazole
tPA	tissue plasminogen activator
TP-HA	*Treponema pallidum* hemagglutination assay
TPP	thiamine pyrophosphate
TRAP	tartrate-resistant acid phosphatase
tRNA	transfer ribonucleic acid
TSH	thyroid-stimulating hormone
TSS	toxic shock syndrome
TTP	thrombotic thrombocytopenic purpura
TURP	transurethral resection of the prostate
TXA	thromboxane A
UA	urinalysis
UDCA	ursodeoxycholic acid
UGI	upper GI
UPPP	uvulopalatopharyngoplasty
URI	upper respiratory infection
US	ultrasound
UTI	urinary tract infection
UV	ultraviolet
VDRL	Venereal Disease Research Laboratory
VIN	vulvar intraepithelial neoplasia
VIP	vasoactive intestinal polypeptide
VLDL	very low density lipoprotein
VMA	vanillylmandelic acid
V/Q	ventilation/perfusion (ratio)
VRE	vancomycin-resistant enterococcus
VS	vital signs
VSD	ventricular septal defect
vWF	von Willebrand factor
VZV	varicella-zoster virus
WAGR	Wilms tumor, aniridia, genitourinary abnormalities, mental retardation (syndrome)
WBC	white blood cell
WHI	Women's Health Initiative
WPW	Wolff-Parkinson-White syndrome
XR	x-ray
ZN	Ziehl-Neelsen (stain)

Underground Clinical Vignettes

Vignettes

Microbiology II: Bacteriology

FIFTH EDITION

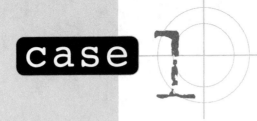

case 1

ID/CC A 54-year-old man presents to his primary care physician with a hard, red, painless **swelling** on his left **mandible** that has slowly been growing over the past few weeks and has now begun to **drain pus.**

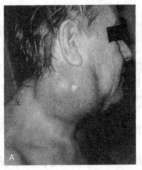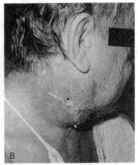

Figure 1-1. Induration and a sinus tract formation with expression of pus.

HPI The patient **recently had a tooth extraction.**

PE No acute distress; no other significant findings.

Labs Gram stain of exudate reveals **branching gram-positive filaments** and characteristic **"sulfur granules"**; non–acid-fast and anaerobic (distinguishes actinomyces from *Nocardia*).

Imaging XR: no bony destruction.

Gross Pathology **Sinus tracts** from region of infection to surface with granular exudate.

Micro Pathology Granulation tissue and fibrosis surrounding a central suppurative necrosis; granulation tissue may also enclose foamy histiocytes and plasma cells.

1

case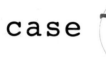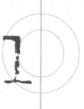

Actinomycosis

Differential

Nocardiosis
Bacterial Abscess
Oral Cavity Cancer
Salivary Gland Cancer
Oral Cutaneous Fistula

Discussion

Actinomyces israelii is a part of the normal flora of the mouth (crypts of tonsils and tartar of teeth), so most patients have a history of surgery or trauma. There is **no person-to-person spread.** Actinomycosis is a chronic suppurative infection and can also involve the abdomen or lungs, especially following a penetrating trauma such as a bullet wound or an intestinal perforation. Pelvic disease is associated with intrauterine device (IUD) use. Spread occurs contiguously, not hematogenously.

Breakout Point

Actinomycetes Infections
Cervicofacial—Most common presentation
Thoracic
Abdominal—Can complicate an appendectomy
Pelvic–Associated with IUD

Treatment

Ampicillin followed by amoxicillin or penicillin G followed by oral penicillin V and, if necessary, surgical drainage and removal of necrotic tissue.

case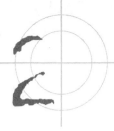

ID/CC   A 25-year-old **IV drug abuser** presents with a **high fever** with chills, malaise, a productive cough, hemoptysis, and right-sided pleuritic chest pain.

HPI   He also reports multiple skin infections at injection sites.

PE   VS: fever. PE: **stigmata of intravenous drug abuse** at multiple injection sites; skin infections; thrombosed peripheral veins; **splenomegaly and pulsatile hepatomegaly; ejection systolic murmur,** increasing with inspiration, heard in the tricuspid area.

Labs   CBC: normochromic, normocytic anemia. UA: microscopic hematuria. Blood culture yields *Staphylococcus aureus.*

Imaging   Echo: presence of **vegetations on tricuspid valve** and **tricuspid incompetence.** CXR: consolidation.

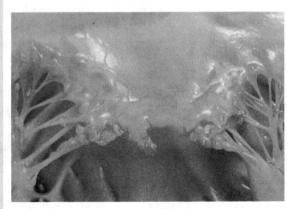

Figure 2-1. Destructive vegetations that have eroded through the free margins of the valve leaflets.

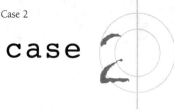

case 2

Acute Bacterial Endocarditis

Differential

Connective Tissue Disease
Septic Pulmonary Infarction
Sepsis
Fever of Unknown Origin
HIV Infection
Tuberculosis

Discussion

In drug addicts, the **tricuspid valve** is the site of infection more frequently (55%) than the aortic valve (35%) or the mitral valve (30%); these findings contrast markedly with the rarity of right-sided involvement in cases of infective endocarditis that are not associated with drug abuse. *Staphylococcus aureus* is responsible for the majority of. Certain organisms have a predilection for particular valves in cases of addict-associated endocarditis; for example, enterococci, other streptococcal species, and non-albicans *Candida* organisms predominantly affect the valves of the left side of the heart, while *S. aureus* infects valves on both the right and the left side of the heart. *Pseudomonas* organisms are associated with biventricular and multiple-valve infection in addicts. Complications of endocarditis include congestive heart failure, ruptured valve cusp, myocardial infarction, and myocardial abscess.

Treatment

High-dose intravenous penicillinase-resistant penicillin in combination with an **aminoglycoside.** If the isolated *S. aureus* strain is **methicillin resistant, vancomycin** is the drug of choice.

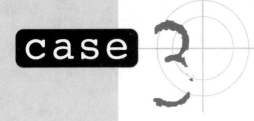

ID/CC A **7-month-old** girl is brought to the pediatric clinic with **wheezing**, respiratory difficulty, and nasal congestion of 3 hours' duration.

HPI She has had rhinorrhea, fever, and cough and had been sneezing for 2 days prior to her visit to the clinic.

PE VS: **tachypnea.** PE: **nasal flaring;** mild central **cyanosis;** accessory muscle use during respiration; hyperexpansion of chest; expiratory and inspiratory wheezes; **rhonchi** over both lung fields.

Labs CBC/PBS: relative **lymphocytosis.** ABGs: **hypoxemia with mild hypercapnia. Respiratory syncytial virus (RSV)** demonstrated on viral culture of throat swab.

Imaging CXR: **hyperinflation;** segmental **atelectasis; interstitial infiltrates.**

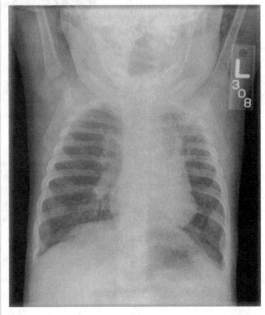

Figure 3-1. Hyperinflation, air trapping, and hilar prominence with peribronchial thickening.

5

case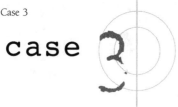

Acute Bronchiolitis

Differential

Asthma
Foreign Body Ingestion
Aspiration Pneumonia
Viral Pneumonia
Bacterial Pneumonia
Congestive Heart Failure

Discussion

RSV is the most common cause of bronchiolitis in infants under 2 years of age; other viral causes include parainfluenza, influenza, and adenovirus. RSV shedding may last 2 or more weeks in children.

Breakout Point

Major Causes of Bronchiolitis in Children
Respiratory Syncytial Virus
Parainfluenza Virus
Adenovirus
Mycoplasma pneumoniae

Treatment

Humidified oxygen, bronchodilators, aerosolized **ribavirin**.

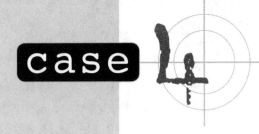

ID/CC A 25-year-old woman visits her family physician because of marked **burning pain while urinating** (DYSURIA), **increased frequency of urination** with **small amounts of urine** (POLLAKIURIA), and passage of a few drops of **blood-stained** debris at the end of urination (HEMATURIA).

HPI She got married 2 weeks ago and has **just returned from her honeymoon.**

PE VS: no fever; BP normal. PE: no edema; no costovertebral angle tenderness; moderate suprapubic tenderness with **urgency.**

Labs UA: urine collected in two glasses; second glass more turbid and blood-stained; urine sediment reveals RBCs and WBCs; **no RBC or WBC casts;** Gram stain of urine sediment reveals **gram-negative bacilli;** *Escherichia coli* in significant colony count (>100,000) on urine culture.

case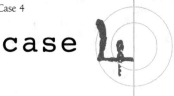

Acute Cystitis

Differential

Endometriosis

Pelvic Inflammatory Disease

Chemical Cystitis

Vaginitis

Herpes Genitalis

Urethral Diverticulum

Discussion

E. coli is the most common pathogen; *Proteus, Klebsiella, Staphylococcus saprophyticus,* and *Enterococcus* are other common bacteria causing cystitis. Hemorrhagic cystitis may result from adenoviral infection.

Treatment

Oral antibiotics (trimethoprim-sulfamethoxazole, fluoroquinolone); adequate hydration.

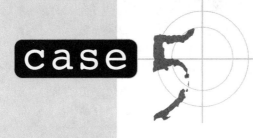

ID/CC An **8-year-old** girl presents with pain and swelling of her knee joints, elbows, and lower limbs along with **fever** for the past 2 weeks; she also complains of shortness of breath (DYSPNEA) on exertion.

HPI The patient had a **sore throat 2 weeks ago.**

PE VS: fever. PE: **blanching, ring-shaped erythematous rash over the trunk and proximal extremities** (ERYTHEMA MARGINATUM); **subcutaneous nodules** at the occiput and below extensor tendons in the elbow; **swelling with redness of both knee joints and elbows** (POLYARTHRITIS); painfully restricted movement; pedal edema; increased JVP; high-frequency apical systolic murmur with radiation to axillae **(mitral valve insufficiency due to carditis);** bilateral fine inspiratory basal crepitant rales; mild, tender hepatomegaly.

Labs CBC: leukocytosis. *Streptococcus pyogenes* on throat swab; markedly **elevated ASO titers; elevated ESR; elevated C-reactive protein (CRP);** negative blood culture. ECG: **prolonged PR interval.**

Imaging CXR: cardiomegaly; increased pulmonary vascular markings. Echo: vegetations over mitral valve with regurgitation.

Gross Pathology Acute form characterized by **endo-, myo-, and pericarditis** (PANCARDITIS); chronic form characterized by fibrous scarring with calcification and mitral stenosis with verrucous fibrin deposits.

Micro Pathology Myocardial muscle fiber necrosis enmeshed in collagen; characteristic finding is fibrinoid necrosis surrounded by **perivascular accumulation of mononuclear inflammatory cells** (ASCHOFF CELLS).

case 5

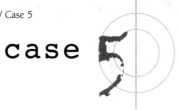

Acute Rheumatic Fever

Differential
Infectious Mononucleosis
Peritonsillar Abscess
Viral Pharyngitis
Kawasaki Disease

Discussion
Acute rheumatic fever is a sequela of upper respiratory infection with group A, β-hemolytic streptococci; it causes **autoimmune** damage to several organs, primarily the heart. The systemic effects of acute rheumatic fever are immune-mediated and are secondary to cross-reactivity of host antistreptococcal antibodies.

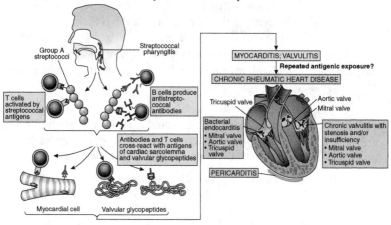

Figure 5-1. Pathogenesis of rheumatic heart disease.

Breakout Point

Jones Criteria for Rheumatic Fever	
JONES crITERIA:	**Minor criteria:**
Major criteria:	Inflammatory cells (leukocytosis)
Joint (arthritis)	**T**emperature (fever)
Obvious (cardiac)	ESR/CRP elevated
Nodule (rheumatic)	**R**aised PR interval
Erythema marginatum	**I**tself (previous history of rheumatic fever)
Sydenham chorea	**A**rthralgia

Treatment
Penicillin to eradicate streptococcal infection; high-dose salicylates for analgesic and anti-inflammatory effect; rest and corticosteroids if there is evidence of carditis resulting in congestive failure; long-term penicillin prophylaxis.

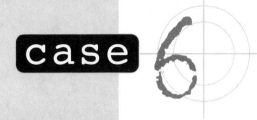
ID/CC	A 35-year-old woman complains of fever and **pain in the face** and **upper teeth** (maxillary sinus), especially while leaning forward.
HPI	She has had a chronic cough, **nasal congestion, and discharge** for the past few months.
PE	VS: fever. PE: halitosis; greenish-yellow **postnasal discharge**; bilateral **boggy nasal mucosa**; bilateral percussion tenderness and **erythema over zygomatic arch; clouding of sinuses by transillumination**; dental and cranial nerve exams normal.
Labs	Nasal cultures reveal *Streptococcus pneumoniae*.
Imaging	CT, sinus: partial opacification of maxillary sinus with air-fluid level.

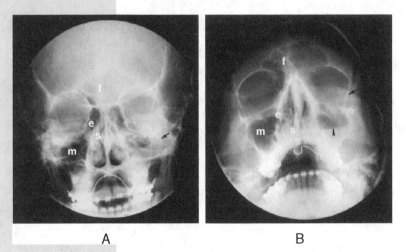

Figure 6-1. There is an air-fluid level in the left maxillary sinus (*arrowhead*) as well as infraorbital soft tissue swelling (*arrow*).

Gross Pathology	Erythematous and edematous nasal mucosa.
Micro Pathology	Presence of organisms and leukocytes in mucosa.

11

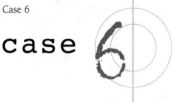

case 6

Acute Sinusitis

Differential

Kartagener Syndrome

Mucormycosis

Allergic Rhinitis

Rhinovirus Infection

Wegener Granulomatosis

Discussion

Other pathogens include other streptococci, *Haemophilus influenzae*, and *Moraxella*. The obstruction of ostia in the anterior ethmoid and middle meatal complex by retained secretions, mucosal edema, or polyps promotes sinusitis. *Staphylococcus aureus* and gram-negative species may cause chronic sinusitis. Fungal sinusitis may mimic chronic bacterial sinusitis. Complications include orbital cellulitis and abscesses.

Treatment

Oral decongestants; amoxicillin, trimethoprim-sulfamethoxazole, or fluoroquinolone.

case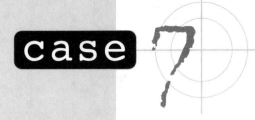

ID/CC   A 30-year-old man goes to the emergency room because of **dyspnea**, cyanosis, hemoptysis, and chest pain.

HPI   He has had a high fever, malaise, and a **nonproductive cough** for 1 week. The patient is a **sheep farmer** who remembers having been treated for **dark black skin lesions** in the past.

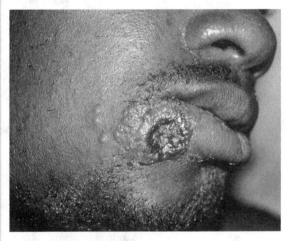

Figure 7-1. Eschar on the face.

PE   VS: fever. PE: dyspnea; cyanosis; bilateral rales heard over the lungs.

Labs   CBC: normal. Negative blood and sputum cultures.

Imaging   CXR: mediastinal widening. CT, chest: evidence of **"hemorrhagic mediastinitis."**

Gross Pathology   Patchy consolidation; vesicular papules covered by **black eschar.**

Micro Pathology   Lungs show fibrinous exudate with many organisms but few PMNs.

13

case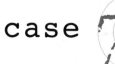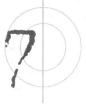

Anthrax

Differential

Coccidioidomycosis

Diphtheria

Lung Abscess

Aortic Dissection

Bronchogenic Carcinoma

Discussion

Anthrax is caused by infection with **Bacillus anthracis.** A cell-free anthrax vaccine is available to protect those employed in industries associated with a high risk of anthrax transmission (farmers, veterinarians, tannery or wool workers). This organism is a potentially lethal organism employed as an agent of **bioterrorism/biological warfare.**

Breakout Point

Potential Bioterrorism Organisms
Bacillus anthracis
Clostridium botulinum
Brucella spp.
Ebola Virus
Franciscella tularensis
Marburg Virus
Rickettsia prowazekii
Salmonella typhi
Shigella spp.
Smallpox Virus
Yersinia pestis

Treatment

Isolate and treat with IV penicillin G, doxycycline, or fluoroquinolones; antibiotics for postexposure prophylaxis of contacts.

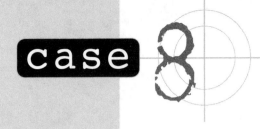

ID/CC A 50-year-old **alcoholic man** presents with a high-grade **fever, cough, copious, foul-smelling sputum,** and pleuritic right-sided chest pain.

HPI His wife reports that he was brought home in a **semi-conscious state a few days ago,** when he was found lying on the roadside heavily under the influence of alcohol.

PE VS: fever. PE: signs of consolidation elicited over the **right middle and lower pulmonary lobes.**

Labs Sputum reveals abundant PMN leukocytes and mixed oral flora; **culture yields *Bacteroides melaninogenicus* (*Prevotella melaninogenica*) and other *Bacteroides* species, *Fusobacterium*, microaerophilic streptococci,** and *Peptostreptococcus.*

Imaging CXR: **consolidation involving apical segment of right lower lobe and posterior segments of middle lobe;** large cavity with air-fluid level also seen.

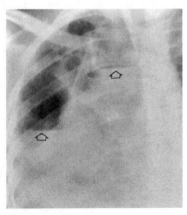

Figure 8-1. Air-fluid levels (*arrows*).

case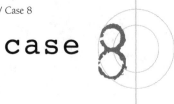

Aspiration Pneumonia with Abscess

Differential

Tracheal Foreign Body

Bronchogenic Carcinoma

Empyema

Sepsis

Community-Acquired Pneumonia

Discussion

Alcoholism, drug abuse, administration of sedatives or anesthesia, head trauma, and seizures or other neurologic disorders are most often responsible for the development of aspiration pneumonia. Because anaerobes are the dominant flora of the upper GI tract (outnumbering aerobic or facultative bacteria by 10 to 1), they are the dominant organisms in aspiration pneumonia; of particular importance are *Bacteroides melaninogenicus* (*Prevotella melaninogenica*) and other *Bacteroides* species (slender, pleomorphic, pale gram-negative rods), *Fusobacterium nucleatum* (slender gram-negative rods with pointed ends), and anaerobic or microaerophilic streptococci and *Peptostreptococcus* (small gram-positive cocci in chains or clumps).

Treatment

Clindamycin.

case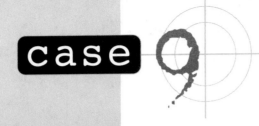

ID/CC A 38-year-old **HIV-positive** man is admitted to the hospital with **fever, rigors, night sweats, and diarrhea.**

HPI He reports excessive weight loss over the past few weeks. He was treated for *Pneumocystis* pneumonia a few weeks ago and still reports a persistent productive cough.

PE VS: fever. PE: patient is extremely emaciated; hepatosplenomegaly and lymphadenopathy noted.

Labs CD4+ count <50/mL; **acid-fast bacilli** are isolated on blood culture; smears of tissues obtained from lymph nodes, bone marrow, spleen, liver, and lungs reveal evidence of acid-fast bacilli.

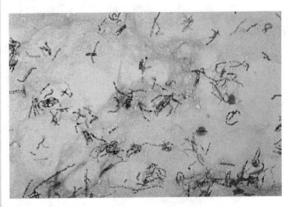

Figure 9-1. Needle aspirate of a lesion on an immunocompromised patient. Abundant elongated and beaded acid-fast bacilli.

Imaging CT, abdomen: hepatosplenomegaly; retroperitoneal lymphadenopathy; bowel mucosal fold thickening.

Micro Pathology Despite the presence of many mycobacteria and macrophages, well-formed granulomas were typically absent due to **profound impairment of cell-mediated immunity.**

17

case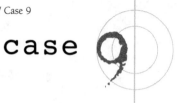

Atypical Mycobacterial Infection

Differential

Cellulitis

Sepsis

Sarcoidosis

Pyoderma Gangrensoum

Actinomycosis

Tuberculosis

Discussion

Mycobacterium avium complex is now the **most frequent opportunistic bacterial infection in patients with AIDS**; it typically occurs late in the course of the syndrome, when other opportunistic infections and neoplasia have already occurred. Prophylaxis against *M. avium-intracellulare* is recommended in AIDS patients with a CD4+ count of <100/mm³ (administer azithromycin, clarithromycin, or rifabutin).

Treatment

Multiagent antibiotic therapy combining one macrolide (e.g., clarithromycin) with ethambutol, rifampin, clofazimine, or quinolones.

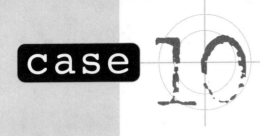

ID/CC A 20-year-old man from **India** presents to the ER with **severe nausea and vomiting.**

HPI Careful history reveals that 2 hours ago he ate some **unrefrigerated fried rice** that his wife had cooked the night before. He does not complain of any fever or diarrhea (may or may not be present).

PE VS: no fever. PE: mild dehydration; diffuse mild abdominal tenderness.

Labs Fecal staining reveals no RBCs, WBCs, or parasites; **a gram-positive rod,** is isolated from vomitus and stool and shown to produce the **emetogenic enterotoxin.**

case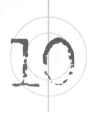

Bacillus cereus Food Poisoning

Differential

Appendicitis

Giardiasis

Salmonella Infection

Staphylococcus aureus Food Poisoning

Clostridial Food Poisoning

Dehydration

Discussion

Bacillus cereus causes two distinct syndromes: a **diarrheal form** (mediated by an *Escherichia coli* LT-type enterotoxin with an incubation period of 8 to 16 hours; caused by meats and vegetables) and an **emetic form** (mediated by a *S. aureus*–type enterotoxin with an incubation period of 1 to 8 hours; caused by fried rice). Proper food handling and refrigeration of boiled rice are largely preventive.

Breakout Point

Common Causes of Food Poisoning
***V**omit **B**ig **S**melly **C**hunks:* ***V**ibrio* ***B**acillus cereus* ***S**taphylococcus aureus* ***C**lostridium perfringens*

Treatment

Supportive.

case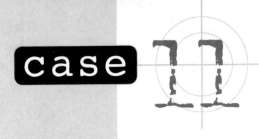

ID/CC A 25-year-old **recently married woman** is concerned about a scanty, offensively **malodorous vaginal discharge.**

HPI She states that the discharge is **thin, grayish-white, and foul-smelling.** She does not complain of vulvar pruritus or soreness.

PE Pelvic exam confirms presence of a homogenous, grayish-white, watery discharge adherent to the vaginal walls that yields a **"fishy" odor when mixed with KOH**; no injection and excoriation of the vulva, vagina, or cervix.

Labs Vaginal pH >5; saline smear reveals presence of **characteristic "clue cells"** (squamous epithelial cells with smudged borders due to adherent bacteria).

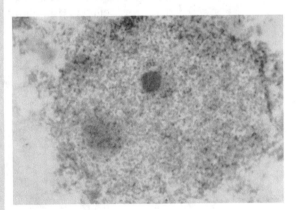

Figure 11-1. Epithelial cell covered with bacteria.

21

case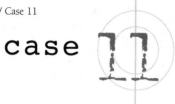

Bacterial Vaginosis

Differential

Cervicitis

Cystitis

Herpes Simplex

Paget Disease

Discussion

Although bacterial vaginitis was originally thought to be caused by *Gardnerella vaginalis*, this organism is now recognized to be part of the normal vaginal flora. Bacterial vaginosis is now known to result from a **synergistic interaction of bacteria** in which the normal *Lactobacillus* species in the vagina is ultimately replaced by **high concentrations of anaerobic bacteria**, including ***Bacteroides, Peptostreptococcus, Peptococcus,*** and ***Mobiluncus* species**, along with a markedly greater number of **G. *vaginalis*** organisms than is encountered in normal vaginal secretions. Bacterial vaginosis is known to increase the risk of pelvic inflammatory disease, chorioamnionitis, and premature birth.

Treatment

A single dose of **metronidazole** (2 g) is effective in treating the infection. Oral clindamycin is an alternative drug.

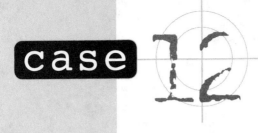

case 12

ID/CC   A 30-year-old man who recently emigrated from **Peru** presents with an extensive **nodular skin eruption**, mild arthralgias, and occasional fever.

HPI   One month ago, the patient had a high-grade **fever** that was accompanied by excessive weakness, dyspnea, and passage of **cola-colored urine**; the fever subsided after 2 weeks, but his weakness has progressed since that time.

PE   Pallor; mild icterus; extensive skin rash comprising **purplish nodular lesions** of varying sizes seen on face, trunk, and limbs; mild hepatosplenomegaly; funduscopy reveals **retinal hemorrhages.**

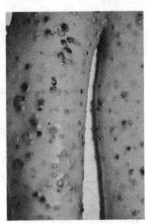

Figure 12-1. Multiple angiomatous lesions on the limbs.

Labs   **Intraerythrocytic coccobacillary**-form bacteria visible in thick and thin films stained with Giemsa; **bacteria** seen and **isolated from skin lesions**; indirect serum bilirubin elevated. PBS: macrocytic, hypochromic anemia with polychromasia; marked reticulocytosis (due to hemolytic anemia); Coombs' test negative.

Micro Pathology   Skin biopsy of vascular skin lesions reveals endothelial proliferation and histiocytic hyperplasia.

23

case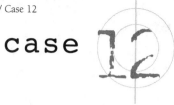

Bartonellosis

Differential

Bacillary Angiomatosis

Lymphoma

Plague

Lymphogranuloma Venereum

Leukemia

Syphilis

Discussion

Bartonellosis is a sandfly-borne bacterial disease occurring only on the **western coast of South America** at high altitudes; the causative agent is a motile, pleomorphic bacillus, *Bartonella bacilliformis*. Two stages of the disease are recognized: an **initial febrile stage** associated with a **hemolytic anemia** (OROYA FEVER), and a later cutaneous stage characterized by **hemangiomatous nodules** (VERRUGA PERUANA).

Breakout Point

Bacterial Pathogens Transmitted by Arthropod Vectors
• *Yersinia pestis*
• *Borrelia recurrentis*
• *Borrelia burgdorferi*
• *Bartonella bacilliformis*

Treatment

Penicillin, erythromycin, norfloxacin, and **tetracycline** are effective; rifampicin is indicated for treatment of verrucous forms.

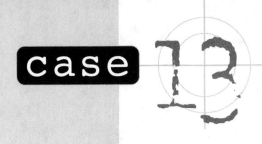

ID/CC A 25-year-old man presents with sudden-onset **double vision** (DIPLOPIA), **dry mouth, weakness, dysarthria,** and **dysphagia.**

HPI He has no previous history of episodic weakness or of dog or tick bites (excluding myasthenia gravis, rabies, or Lyme disease). Last night, he ate some **home-canned food.**

PE VS: no fever. PE: patient alert; ptosis; bilateral **third and tenth cranial nerve palsy;** symmetric **flaccid paralysis** of all four limbs; deep tendon reflexes reduced; no sensory loss seen; decreased bowel sounds.

Labs Botulinum toxin detected in patient's serum and canned-food sample with specific antiserum.

case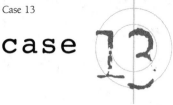

Botulism

Differential

Hypermagnesemia
Hyperthyroidism
Myasthenia Gravis
Guillain-Barré Syndrome
Lambert-Eaton Syndrome
Poliomyelitis

Discussion

The disease is characterized by gradual return of muscle strength in most cases. Botulinum toxin is a zinc metalloprotease that cleaves specific components of synaptic vesicle docking and fusion complexes, thus **inhibiting the release of acetylcholine at the neuromuscular junction.** The disease in adults is due to **ingestion of the toxin** rather than to bacterial infection. Botulism is also seen in infants secondary to the ingestion of *Clostridium botulinum* spores in **honey.**

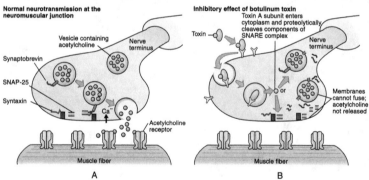

Figure 13-1. Mechanism of action of botulinum toxins.

Treatment

Antitoxin; close monitoring of respiratory status; intubation for respiratory failure.

Breakout Point

Bacterial Infections for Which Antitoxins are used
• *Corynebacterium diphtheriae*
• *Corynebacterium botulinum*
• *Clostridium tetani*

ID/CC A 10-year-old girl presents with a **high fever, headache, vomiting,** and impaired consciousness.

HPI She suffered a generalized **seizure** about 45 minutes ago. She was previously diagnosed with **cyanotic congenital heart disease** (ventricular septal defect with Eisenmenger's syndrome).

PE VS: fever. PE: altered sensorium; **papilledema;** nuchal rigidity; clubbing; **central cyanosis;** cardiac auscultation suggestive of VSD with severe pulmonary arterial hypertension.

Labs Blood culture reveals **mixed infection.**

Imaging CT (with contrast): ring-enhancing lesion with low attenuation center surrounding cerebral edema and ventricular compression.

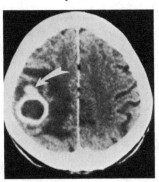

Figure 14-1. Contrast-enhanced study shows a thick but uniformly enhancing capsule with the beginnings of a daughter lesion anteriorly (*arrow*).

Gross Pathology Cavity filled with thick, liquefied pus surrounded by fibrous capsule of variable thickness; pericapsular zone of gliosis and edema.

Micro Pathology Central portion contains degenerated PMNs and cellular debris; capsule is composed of collagenous fibrous tissue with blood vessels and mixed inflammatory cells.

27

case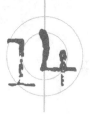

Brain Abscess

Differential

Venous Sinus Thrombosis
Cryptococcosis
Cysticercosis
Toxoplasmosis
Metastatic Tumor
Primary CNS Neoplasm

Breakout Point

> ### Major Differential Diagnosis of a Ring Enhancing Cerebral Mass
> - Brain Abscess
> - Toxoplasmosis
> - Glioblastoma Multiforme

Discussion

Brain abscesses arise secondary to **hematogenous spread** from another infection (bronchiectasis, endocarditis), from contiguous spread from adjacent infection (chronic otitis media, mastoiditis, sinusitis), or following **direct implantation** from trauma. Often they are **mixed infections** with *Bacteroides,* microaerophilic streptococci, *Staphylococcus aureus,* and *Klebsiella.* Patients with congenital heart disease with right-to-left shunt are particularly predisposed because the normal filtering action of the pulmonary vasculature is lost.

Treatment

High-dose, extended parenteral broad-spectrum antibiotic coverage; **CT-directed drainage of pus.**

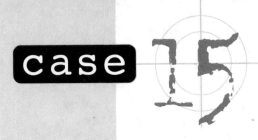
ID/CC A 25-year-old puerpera who was **lactating** to feed her week-old infant presents with **pain and swelling** in her left breast.

HPI The symptoms commenced acutely, and she does not recall any previous breast lumps or swellings.

PE **Skin overlying** the left breast is **red, edematous, tender, and hot;** area of tense induration felt underlying inflamed skin.

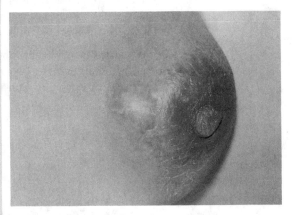

Figure 15-1. Edematous area of tense induration.

Labs Culture of pus drained **grew Staphylococcus aureus.**

Imaging USG: nearly anechoic area with posterior enhancement.

case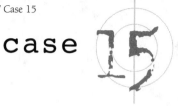

Breast Abscess

Differential

Cellulitis
Fibroadenoma
Fibrocystic Disease
Breast Cancer
Fat Necrosis
Mastitis

Discussion

Bacterial mastitis most commonly occurs in lactating women due to infection of a hematoma or secondary infection of plasma cell mastitis; the infecting **organism is mostly penicillin-resistant** *Staphylococcus aureus.*

Treatment

Penicillinase-resistant antibiotic; incision (in a radial direction over the affected segment) **and dependent drainage** of intramammary abscess; patient may continue nursing from the affected breast.

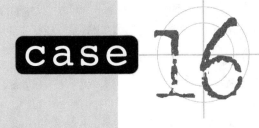

case 16

ID/CC A 28-year-old white man visits his family doctor complaining of acute **pain in both hip joints** together with weakness, backache, myalgias, arthralgias, and **undulating fever** of **2 months' duration**; this morning he woke up with pain in his right testicle.

HPI For the past 3 years he has worked at the largest dairy farm in his state. He enjoys **drinking "crude" milk**.

PE VS: fever. PE: pallor; marked pain on palpation of sacroiliac joints; mild splenomegaly; generalized lymphadenopathy.

Labs CBC: relative lymphocytosis with normal WBC count.

Imaging XR, hips: joint effusion and soft tissue swelling without destruction. MR, spine: evidence of spondylitis.

Gross Pathology Lymphadenopathy and splenomegaly; hepatomegaly rare.

Micro Pathology Granulomatous foci in spleen, liver, and lymph nodes, with proliferation of macrophages; epithelioid and giant cells may be seen.

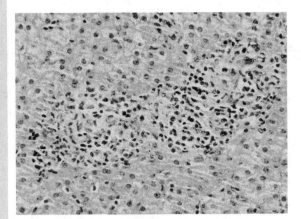

Figure 16-1. Nonspecific lymphoplasmacytic inflammatory infiltrate in the liver of the patient.

31

case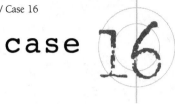

Brucellosis

Differential

Ankylosing Spondylitis

Leptospirosis

Tuberculosis

Cryptococcosis

Typhoid Fever

Discussion

Also called Malta fever, a microbial disease of animals, brucellosis is caused by several species of *Brucella*, a gram-negative, aerobic coccobacillus. It is transmitted to humans through the drinking of contaminated milk or through direct contact with products or tissues from animals such as goats, sheep, camels, cows, hogs, and dogs. The clinical picture is often vague; thus, a high index of suspicion may be necessary for diagnosis.

Breakout Point

Bacterial Diseases Associated with the Consumption of Milk Products
• *Brucella*
• *Listeria*
• *Streptobacillus moniliformis*
• *Mycobacterium bovis*
• *Escherichia coli*
• *Yersinia enterocolitica*

Treatment

Combination therapy with doxycycline or TMP-SMX and rifampin or streptomycin.

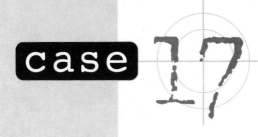

ID/CC   A 26-year-old woman presents to the ER with intense, acute-onset left **lower quadrant crampy abdominal pain,** foul-smelling stools with streaks of blood, urgency, **tenesmus,** and fever.

HPI   For the past 2 days, the patient has also had headaches and myalgias. She frequently **drinks unpasteurized** ("raw") **milk** that she buys at a health-food store.

PE   VS: fever (39°C); tachycardia; normal RR and BP. PE: no dehydration; diffuse abdominal tenderness more marked in left lower quadrant.

Labs   Stool smear shows leukocytes (due to invasive tissue damage in the colon) and **gram-negative, curved bacilli,** often in pairs, in "gull-wing"–shaped pattern.

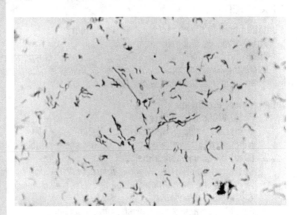

Figure 17-1. Curved, "gull wing"–shaped organism.

Gross Pathology   Friable colonic mucosa.

Micro Pathology   Nonspecific inflammatory reaction consisting of neutrophils, lymphocytes, and plasma cells with hyperemia, edema, and damage to epithelium, glandular degeneration, ulcerations, and crypt abscesses caused by colonic tissue invasion of the organism.

case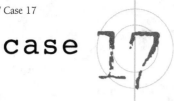

Campylobacter Enteritis

Differential	Arteriovenous Malformation
	Clostridium difficile Colitis
	Inflammatory Bowel Disease
	Mesenteric Artery Ischemia
	Shigellosis
	Yersinia enterocolitica
Discussion	One of the primary causes of "traveler's diarrhea." Sources of infection include **undercooked food** and contact with **infected animals** and their excreta. Prevent by improving public sanitation, pasteurizing milk, and proper cooking.

■ **TABLE 17-1 FECAL LEUKOCYTES IN ACUTE DIARRHEAL DISORDERS**

Noninflammatory diarrheas: fecal WBCs absent
  Viral: rotavirus, Norwalk agent
  Protozoal: *Giardia, Cryptosporidium, Cyclospora, Isospora*
  Bacterial: *Staphylococcus aureus, Bacillus cereus, Clostridium perfringens,* enterotoxigenic *Escherichia coli, Vibrio cholerae*

Inflammatory diarrheas
  1. **Fecal WBCs usually present**
    Bacterial: *Shigella, Campylobacter jejuni* •
    Noninfectious: ulcerative colitis, Crohn disease, radiation or ischemic colitis
  2. **Fecal WBCs variably present**
    Bacterial: *Salmonella, Yersinia enterocolitica, Vibrio parahaemolyticus, Aeromonas, Listeria monocytogenes, Escherichia coli* O157:H7, *Clostridium difficile*
  3. **Fecal WBCs absent:** amebiasis, cytomegalovirus

WBC, white blood cell.

Treatment	Fluid and electrolyte replacement; macrolides (e.g., erythromycin) for persistent or severe disease.

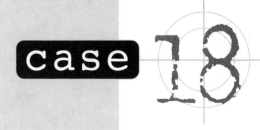

ID/CC A 14-year-old girl presents with **painful lumps in her right axilla** and neck, together with **low-grade fever.**

HPI Three weeks ago she was **scratched** on her right forearm **by her pet cat;** an erythematous pustule initially developed at the site but resolved spontaneously within 10 days.

PE VS: fever. PE: **tender right axillary** and cervical **lymphadenopathy.**

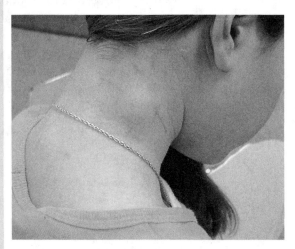

Figure 18-1. Posterior cervical adenopathy in the patient.

Labs Lymph node biopsy diagnostic.

Micro Pathology Hematoxylin and eosin staining reveals **granulomatous pathology** with stellate necrosis and surrounding palisades of histiocytic cells; **Warthin–Starry silver stain** reveals **clumps of pleomorphic, strongly argyrophilic bacilli.**

case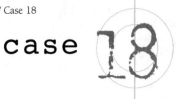

Cat-Scratch Disease

Differential
Brucellosis
Plague
Lymphogranuloma Venereum
Mononucleosis
Sarcoidosis
Tularemia

Discussion
Bartonella henselae is the agent that causes cat-scratch disease. Lymphadenopathy can persist for months and can sometimes be mistaken for a malignancy. Individuals who are immunocompromised may present with seizures, coma, and meningitis.

Treatment
Disease is usually self-limited in immunocompetent hosts; immunocompromised patients may need antibiotic treatment with rifampin, ciprofloxacin, TMP-SMX, or gentamicin.

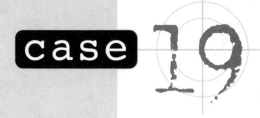

ID/CC A 54-year-old woman who **underwent** a left mastectomy with **axillary lymph node dissection** a year ago presents with **pain** together with rapidly spreading **redness** and **swelling** of the left **arm**.

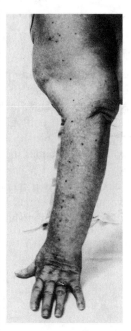

Figure 19-1. Swelling and erythema of left arm in this patient.

HPI One year ago, she was diagnosed and operated on for stage 1 **carcinoma of the left breast**.

PE Left forearm swollen, indurated, pink, and markedly tender; overlying temperature raised; margins and borders of skin lesion ill-defined and not elevated (excludes erysipelas).

Labs Needle aspiration from advancing border of the lesion, when stained and cultured, shows isolated **β-hemolytic group A** streptococci.

case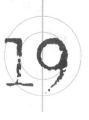

Cellulitis

Differential

Impetigo
Partial-Thickness Burn
Osteomyelitis
Dermatitis
Erysipelas
Ecthyma

Discussion

Cellulitis is an acute spreading infection of the skin that predominantly affects deeper subcutaneous tissue. **Group A streptococci and** *Staphylococcus aureus* are the **most common** etiologic agents in adults; *Haemophilus influenzae* infection is common in children. Patients with chronic venous stasis and lymphedema of any cause (lymphoma, filariasis, post-regional lymph node dissection, radiation therapy) are predisposed; recently, recurrent saphenous vein donor-site cellulitis was found to be attributable to group A, C, or G streptococci.

Treatment

Penicillinase-resistant penicillin (nafcillin/oxacillin).

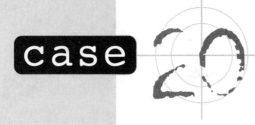

ID/CC A 30-year-old man has sudden severe, **profuse (several liters per day) watery diarrhea, protracted vomiting,** and **abdominal pain.**

HPI He is a resident of a refugee camp in **rural India.**

PE **Severe dehydration;** low urine output; generalized mild abdominal tenderness with no signs of peritoneal irritation; stools have characteristic **"rice-water" appearance** (gray, slightly cloudy fluid with flecks of mucus), with no blood.

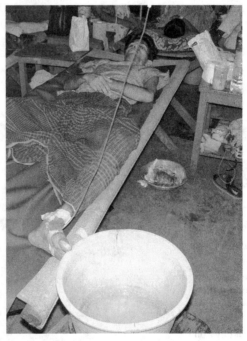

Figure 20-1. Patient excreting large volumes of nonbloody rice-water stool.

Labs Stool culture reveals gram-negative rods with **"darting motility"; O1 antigen detected;** serum chloride levels decreased; serum sodium levels increased.

case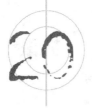

Cholera

Differential

Salmonellosis
Giardiasis
Irritable Bowel Syndrome
Rotavirus Infection
Escherichia coli (*E. coli*) Infection (Enterotoxigenic)

Discussion

A heat-labile exotoxin produced by *Vibrio cholerae* that acts by permanently **stimulating G_S protein via ADP ribosylation,** resulting in activation of **intracellular adenylate cyclase,** which in turn increases cAMP levels and produces **secretory diarrhea.**

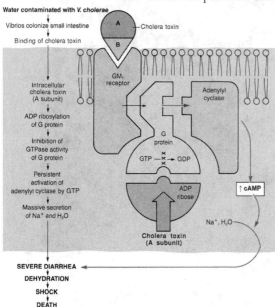

Figure 20-2. Mechanism of action of *Vibrio cholerae.* ADP, adenosine diphosphate; cAMP, cyclic adenosine monophosphate; GDP, guanosine diphosphate; GTP, guanosine triphosphate.

Breakout Point

Bacterial Virulence Factors that Interfere with cAMP- or Cyclic Guanosine Monophosphate (cGMP)-Mediated Signaling	
• *Bacillus anthracis*	• *E. coli* ST **toxin**
• *Vibrio cholerae*	• *Bordetella pertussis*
• *E. coli* LT **toxin**	• *Bacillus cereus*

Treatment

Vigorous rehydration therapy with oral and/or IV fluids; **tetracycline,** ciprofloxacin, or doxycycline.

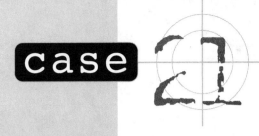

case

ID/CC A 28-year-old primigravida at 36 weeks' gestation presents with a **high fever**.

HPI She was being monitored following a **premature rupture of the membranes**.

PE VS: **fever**; fetal tachycardia. PE: **uterine tenderness**.

Labs Elevated maternal total lymphocyte count; **vaginal swab** culture revealed colonization with **group B streptococci**.

case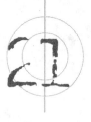

Chorioamnionitis

Differential

Herpes Simplex Infection

Urinary Tract Infection

Vaginitis

Cervicitis

Pelvic Inflammatory Disease

Discussion

A significant proportion of the population is colonized in the vagina and rectum with **group B streptococci, which is correlated with preterm labor, premature rupture of membranes** (PROM), **chorioamnionitis, and neonatal sepsis;** neonates with group B streptococcal sepsis have a 25% mortality rate. Among preterm neonates, this figure doubles to over 50%; therefore **antibiotic prophylaxis** is recommended in the setting of **preterm delivery and PROM,** even without the diagnosis of frank chorioamnionitis. When chorioamnionitis is suspected, intravenous antibiotics are started and delivery is hastened.

Treatment

Presence of group B streptococci in the vagina after premature rupture of membranes was an indication for **immediate delivery and treatment of the infant;** the mother was also treated with an **antibiotic** regimen that included clindamycin, gentamicin, and ampicillin.

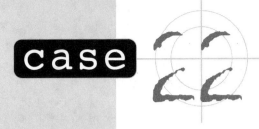

ID/CC A **5-year-old** white boy presents with malaise, anorexia, low-grade fever, sore throat of 3 days' duration, and dyspnea on exertion.

HPI The child was raised abroad. His immunization status cannot be determined.

PE VS: fever; tachycardia with occasional dropped beats. PE: **cervical lymphadenopathy** (BULL-NECK APPEARANCE); smooth, **whitish-gray, adherent membrane over the tonsils and pharynx**; no hepatosplenomegaly; diminished intensity of S_1.

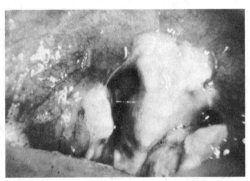

Figure 22-1. Pseudomembranes on the soft palate and uvula.

Labs **Metachromatic granules** in **bacilli arranged in "Chinese character" pattern** on Albert stain of throat culture. ECG: ST-segment elevation; second-degree heart block.

Imaging Echo: evidence of myocarditis.

Gross Pathology Pharyngeal membranes not restricted to anatomic landmarks; pale and enlarged heart.

Micro Pathology Polymorphonuclear exudate with bacteria; precipitated fibrin and cell debris forming a **pseudomembrane**; marked hyperemia, edema, and necrosis of upper respiratory tract mucosa; exotoxin-induced myofibrillar hyaline degeneration; lysis of myelin sheath.

43

case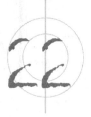

Diphtheria

Differential

Angioedema

Epiglottitis

Mononucleosis

Pharyngitis

Peritonsillar Abscess

Discussion

A bacterial infection of the throat, diphtheria is preventable by vaccine and is caused by toxigenic *Corynebacterium diphtheriae*, a club-shaped, gram-positive aerobic bacillus. Diphtheria toxin is produced by β-prophage-infected corynebacteria; it blocks elongation factor-2 (EF-2) via ADP ribosylation and hence ribosomal function in protein synthesis. The toxin enters the bloodstream, causing **fever**, **myocarditis** (within the first 2 weeks), and **polyneuritis** (many weeks later).

Breakout Point

Corynebacteria Virulence Factor (ABCDEF)
AB Toxin
Corynebacterium
Diphtheria
ADP Ribosylates
Elongation
Factor-2

Treatment

Begin treatment on presumptive diagnosis; specific antitoxin and penicillin or erythromycin; respiratory and cardiac support; confirm eradication by repeating throat culture.

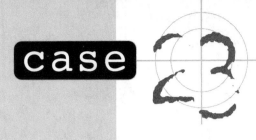

case 23

ID/CC	A 28-year-old man who is a resident of the **south-eastern United States** presents with a high **fever with chills, headache, and myalgias.**
HPI	He remembers having been **bitten by a tick** a week before developing his symptoms; however, he reports no skin rash.
PE	VS: fever. PE: no skin rash noted.
Labs	CBC: leukopenia and mild thrombocytopenia. **Characteristic intraleukocytic inclusion bodies** (MORULAE).

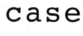 case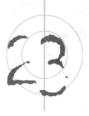

Ehrlichiosis

Differential

Babesiosis

Malaria

Meningitis

Rocky Mountain Spotted Fever

Typhoid Fever

Discussion

Ehrlichia are gram-negative, obligately intracellular bacteria. The two types of *Ehrlichia* species that affect humans are *E. chaffeensis* (which attacks macrophages and monocytes) and an *E. equi*-like organism (which attacks granulocytes). Preventive measures include wearing clothing that covers the body and using insect repellants.

Breakout Point

> ***Ehrlichia chaffeensis*** and ***Borrelia burgdorferi*** (the causative agent of Lyme disease) are both transmitted by the bite of the *Ixodes* tick.

Treatment

Doxycycline.

case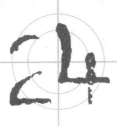

ID/CC A **4-year-old** boy presents with **fever, hoarseness,** and respiratory distress because of partial **airway obstruction.**

HPI The child is also **unable to speak clearly and has pain while swallowing** (ODYNOPHAGIA).

PE VS: fever; tachypnea. PE: **patient is leaning forward with his neck hyperextended and chin protruding; drooling;** marked suprasternal and infrasternal retraction of the chest; **inspiratory stridor** on auscultation.

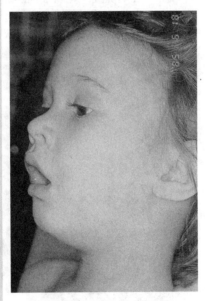

Figure 24-1. Classic sniffing position assumed to maximize patency of the airway.

Labs Culture of throat swab (no role in management of acute disease) reveals penicillinase-resistant *Haemophilus influenzae*; blood cultures also positive.

Imaging XR, neck: marked edema of epiglottis and aryepiglottic folds ("THUMBPRINT" SIGN).

case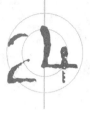

Epiglottitis

Differential

Airway Foreign Body
Bacterial Tracheitis
Croup
Thermal Burns
Laryngomalacia
Peritonsillar Abscess
Retropharyngeal Abscess

Discussion

The principal cause of acute epiglottitis in children and adults is *H. influenzae* type b; other pathogens include *H. parainfluenzae* and group A streptococci. Characterized by rapid onset.

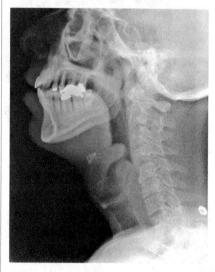

Figure 24-2. Soft tissue radiograph showing thumbprint sign.

Breakout Point

> Since the introduction of the *Haemophilus influenzae* vaccine, the number of cases of epiglottitis has significantly decreased.

Treatment

Preservation of the airway; IV cefuroxime; rifampin prophylaxis for contacts.

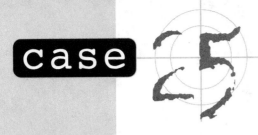

case 25

ID/CC   A 36-year-old African American woman presents to the outpatient clinic with a **painful facial rash** and **fever**.

HPI   One week ago, the patient went on a camping trip and scratched her face on some low-lying tree branches. There is no medical history of diabetes, cancer, or other chronic conditions.

PE   VS: **fever** (39.0°C); tachycardia (HR 110); BP normal. PE: **erythematous, warm, plaquelike rash** extending across cheeks and face bilaterally with **sharp, distinct borders** and **facial swelling**.

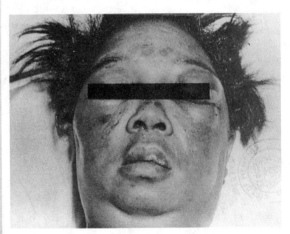

Figure 25-1. Facial erythema and swelling.

Labs   CBC: **leukocytosis** with **neutrophilia. ESR elevated.**

case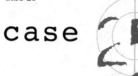

Erysipelas

Differential

Angioedema

Cellulitis

Contact Dermatitis

Necrotizing Fasciitis

Urticaria

Systemic Lupus Erythematosus

Discussion

Erysipelas is an acute inflammation of the superficial layers of the connective tissues of the skin, usually on the face, almost always caused by infection with group A streptococci, which is part of normal bacterial skin flora. Risk factors include any breaks in the skin or **lymphedema.**

Treatment

Antibiotics with sufficient coverage for penicillinase-producing *Streptococcus* and *Staphylococcus* spp. (e.g., cephalexin); **analgesics/antipyretics;** elevate the affected part to reduce swelling.

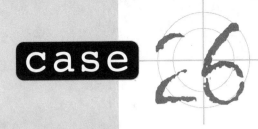

case 26

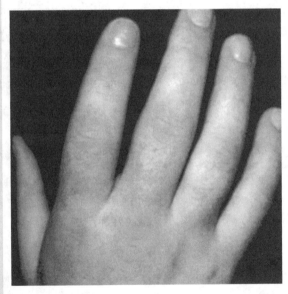

ID/CC   A 30-year-old **fisherman** presents with a **painful red swelling** of the **index finger** of his right hand.

HPI   The swelling developed 4 days after he was **injured** with a knife **while cutting up chum.**

PE   Well-defined, exquisitely tender, slightly elevated **violaceous lesion seen on finger;** no suppuration noted; right epitrochlear and right axillary lymphadenopathy noted.

Figure 26-1. Erythema and induration spreading out radially from the puncture site.

Labs   Biopsy from edge of lesion yields a thin, pleomorphic, nonsporulating, microaerophilic gram-positive rod.

case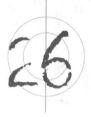

Erysipeloid

Differential

Cellulitis

Erysipelas

Contact Dermatitis

Herpes Zoster

Orf

Discussion

Erysipeloid refers to **localized cellulitis,** usually of the fingers and hands, caused by *Erysipelothrix rhusiopathiae;* infection in humans is usually the result of **contact with infected animals** or their products **(often fish).** Organisms gain entry via cuts and abrasions of the skin.

Breakout Point

Bacterial Infections Associated With Occupational Exposures
• Brucellosis
• Tularemia
• Anthrax
• Erysipeloid

Treatment

Penicillin G; erythromycin and rifampin for patients allergic to penicillin.

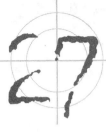

case 27

ID/CC A **30-year-old woman** presents to the surgical ER complaining of a stabbing **right upper quadrant abdominal pain.**

HPI She is a prostitute who has been receiving treatment for **gonococcal pelvic inflammatory disease.**

PE Right upper quadrant tenderness; cervical motion tenderness and mucopurulent cervicitis found on pelvic exam.

Labs Cervical swab staining and culture identifies *Neisseria gonorrhoeae.*

Imaging US: no evidence of cholecystitis. Peritoneoscopy: presence of **"violin string"** adhesions between liver capsule and peritoneum.

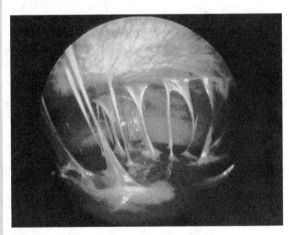

Figure 27-1. Laparoscopic view of violin string adhesions.

Gross Pathology Adhesions noted between liver capsule and peritoneum.

case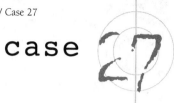

Fitz–Hugh–Curtis Syndrome

Differential
Cholecystitis
Hepatitis
Nephrolithiasis
Pneumonia
Peptic Ulcer Disease

Discussion
Acute fibrinous perihepatitis (FITZ–HUGH–CURTIS SYNDROME) occurs as a complication of **gonococcal and chlamydial pelvic inflammatory disease** and clinically mimics cholecystitis.

Treatment
Antibiotic therapy (ceftriaxone and doxycycline) for patient (and for partner if warranted).

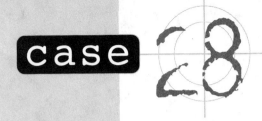

ID/CC A 30-year-old soldier who had been admitted for a **gunshot wound** in the right thigh presents with **severe pain and swelling** at the site of his injury.

HPI The patient's right lower limb had become discolored, and several bullae had appeared on the skin.

PE VS: low-grade fever; marked tachycardia. PE: diaphoresis; skin of right thigh discolored (bronze to purple red); site of injury exquisitely tender and tense and **oozing** a thin, dark, and **foul-smelling fluid; crepitus** while palpating the thigh.

Labs CBC: low hematocrit. Gram stain of exudate and necrotic material at wound site reveals presence of **large gram-positive rods**.

Imaging XR, right thigh: presence of **gas in soft tissues.**

Gross Pathology Overlying skin purple-bronze, markedly edematous with vesiculobullous changes with little suppurative reaction.

Micro Pathology **Coagulative necrosis,** edema, **gas formation,** and many large **gram-positive bacilli** found in affected muscle tissue; relatively sparse infiltration of PMNs noted in the bordering muscle tissue.

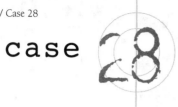

case 28

Gas Gangrene—Traumatic

Differential | Cellulitis
Deep Vein Thrombosis
Necrotizing Fasciitis
Pyoderma Gangrenosum
Drug Reaction

Discussion | A rapidly progressive myonecrosis caused by *Clostridium perfringens* type A, traumatic gas gangrene develops in a wound with low oxygen tension (embedded foreign bodies containing calcium or silicates cause lowering of oxygen tension, leading to germination of the spores). The most important toxin is the alpha toxin lecithinase, which produces hemolysis and myonecrosis.

Treatment | Surgical débridement; antibiotics (penicillin, clindamycin, tetracycline, metronidazole); hyperbaric oxygen therapy and polyvalent antitoxin; supportive management of associated multiorgan failure.

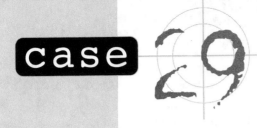
case 29

ID/CC A 25-year-old man presents with sudden-onset, severe **vomiting,** nausea, **abdominal cramps, and diarrhea.**

HPI He had returned home about 2 hours after attending a birthday party at which **meat and milk** were served in various forms. The **friend** who was celebrating his birthday **reported similar symptoms.**

PE VS: **no fever.** PE: mild dehydration; diffuse abdominal tenderness; increased bowel sounds.

Labs **Toxigenic staphylococci** recovered from culturing food. Coagulase-positive staphylococci cultured from the **nose of one of the cooks** at the party.

Micro Pathology No mucosal lesions.

case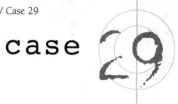

Gastroenteritis—*Staphylococcus aureus*

Differential

Celiac Sprue

Salmonella Food Poisoning

Clostridial Food Poisoning

Viral Gastroenteritis

Short Bowel Syndrome

Diverticulitis

Discussion

Staphylococcus aureus food poisoning results from the ingestion of food containing **preformed heat-stable enterotoxin B.** Outbreaks of staphylococcal food poisoning occur when **food handlers** who have contaminated superficial wounds or who are shedding infected nasal droplets inoculate foods such as meat, dairy products, salad dressings, cream sauces, and custard-filled pastries. The **incubation period** ranges from **2 to 8 hours;** the disease is self-limited.

Treatment

Fluid and electrolyte balance; antibiotics not indicated.

case 30

ID/CC	A **3-day-old** girl presents with a **thick eye discharge.**
HPI	The **mother** admits to having **multiple sexual partners** and complains of a **vaginal discharge.** She did not receive adequate antenatal care.
PE	Exam of both eyes reveals a **thick purulent discharge** and marked **conjunctival congestion** and edema; conjunctival **chemosis** is so marked that cornea is seen at the bottom of a craterlike pit; **corneal ulceration** noted.

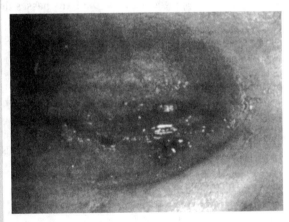

Figure 30-1. Typical purulent discharge.

Labs	Conjunctival swabs on Gram staining reveal presence of **gram-negative diplococci** both intra- and extra-cellularly, in addition to **many PMNs.**

case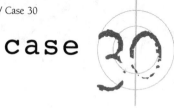

Gonococcal Ophthalmia Neonatorum

Differential

Orbital Cellulitis

Dacryocystitis

Keratitis

Conjunctivitis

Nasolacrimal Duct Obstruction

Trachoma

Discussion

Caused by **Neisseria gonorrhoeae,** gonococcal oph- thalmia neonatorum is **contracted** from a mother with gonorrhea **as the fetus passes down the birth canal;** infection does not occur in utero. **Corneal inflamma- tion** is the major clinical sign that may produce compli- cations such as corneal opacities, perforation, anterior synechiae, anterior staphyloma, and panophthalmitis. It is now common practice to **prevent** this disease by treating the **eyes of the newborn with an antibacter- ial** compound such as erythromycin ointment or 1% silver nitrate; however, home childbirth bypasses this prophylactic procedure, and thus some cases are still occurring in the United States.

Treatment

Penicillin G or **ceftriaxone.** Also treat the mother and her sexual contacts.

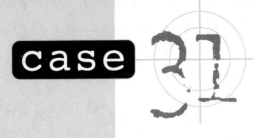
ID/CC A 19-year-old white man presents with **burning urination**; profuse, **greenish-yellow, purulent urethral discharge**; staining of his underwear; and urethral pain.

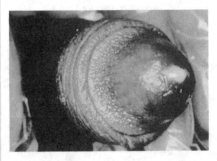

Figure 31-1. Purulent urethral discharge.

HPI Four days ago, he had **unprotected sexual contact** with a prostitute.

PE **Mucopurulent** and slightly blood-tinged urethral discharge; normal testes and epididymis; no urinary retention.

Labs Smear of urethral discharge reveals **intracellular gram-negative diplococci** in WBCs; gonococcal infection confirmed by inoculation into **Thayer-Martin medium**.

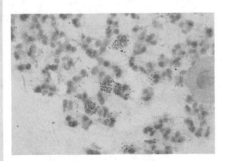

Figure 31-2. Gram-negative diplococci in a urethral specimen.

Gross Pathology Abundant, purulent urethral exudate.

61

case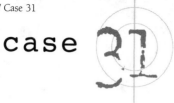

Gonorrhea

Differential

Chlamydia

Urinary Tract Infection

Testicular Torsion

Epididymitis

Orchitis

Discussion

A common STD caused by *Neisseria gonorrhoeae*, gonorrhea may involve the throat, anus, rectum, epididymis, cervix, fallopian tubes, prostate, and joints; conjunctivitis is also found in neonates. Neonatal conjunctivitis may be prevented through the instillation of silver nitrate or erythromycin eye drops at birth.

Breakout Point

Common Culture Media for Select Organisms

- Thayer Martin Media—*Neisseria*
- Chocolate Agar—*Haemophilus*
- Bordet-Gengou Media—*Bordetella*
- Cysteine-Containing media—*Legionella*

Treatment

Ceftriaxone; add doxycycline or erythromycin for **possible coinfection with *Chlamydia*.**

case

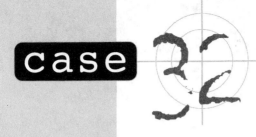

ID/CC A 45-year-old man with refractory **acute myeloid leukemia** who underwent a **bone marrow transplant** from a nonidentical donor presents with an **extensive skin rash**, severe **diarrhea**, and **jaundice**.

HPI Prior to the transplant, which occurred 2 months ago, he **received preparative chemotherapy and radiotherapy** along with broad-spectrum antibiotics. Engraftment was confirmed within 4 weeks by rising leukocyte counts.

PE VS: BP normal. PE: patient is cachectic and moderately dehydrated; icterus noted; violaceous, scaly macules and erythematous papules **resembling lichen planus** seen over the extremities.

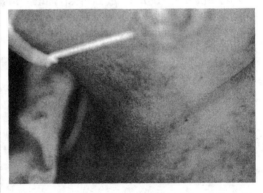

Figure 32-1. Florid papular eruption of the neck and trunk.

Labs CBC: falling blood counts; relative eosinophilia. Elevated direct serum bilirubin and transaminases; stool exam reveals no infectious etiology; skin biopsy taken.

Gross Pathology Skin biopsy specimens reveal vacuolar changes of basal cell layer with perivenular lymphocytic infiltrates (CD8+ T cells).

case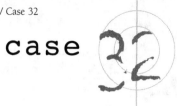

Graft-Versus-Host Disease

Differential

Erythema Multiforme

Stevens–Johnson Syndrome

Mixed Connective Tissue Disease

Scleroderma

Cytomegalovirus Infection

Discussion

Approximately 30% of bone marrow transplant recipients develop graft-versus-host disease (GVHD). This attack is primarily launched by immunocompetent T lymphocytes derived from the donor's marrow against the cells and tissues of the recipient, which it recognizes as foreign. Cyclosporine A is effective for prevention of GVHD.

Treatment

High-dose cyclosporine therapy, anti-thymocyte globulin, methylprednisolone, or anti–T-cell monoclonal antibodies.

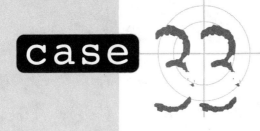

case 33

ID/CC A 28-year-old **immigrant** presents with **inguinal swelling** and a **painless penile ulcer.**

HPI He admits to unprotected intercourse with **multiple sexual partners,** many of whom were prostitutes. He first noticed a papule on his penis several weeks ago.

PE Soft, **painless,** raised, **beefy-red,** smooth **granulating ulcer** noted on distal penis; multiple **subcutaneous swellings** (PSEUDOBUBOES) noted in inguinal region, some of which have ulcerated.

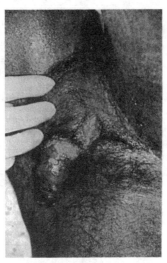

Figure 33-1. Erosion of the base of the penis and inguinal area.

Labs Giemsa-stained smear from penile and inguinal regions demonstrates characteristic **"closed safety pin"** appearance of encapsulated organisms **within a large histiocyte** (DONOVAN BODIES).

Micro Pathology Characteristic histologic picture of donovanosis comprises some degree of epithelial hyperplasia at margins of lesions; dense plasma cell infiltrate scatters histiocyte-containing Donovan bodies.

case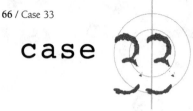

Granuloma Inguinale

Differential

Lymphogranuloma Venereum
Syphilis
Mycobacterial Infection
Herpes Simplex

Discussion

Granuloma inguinale, a slowly progressive, ulcerative, granulomatous STD involving the genitalia, is caused by the gram-negative bacillus ***Calymmatobacterium granulomatis*** (formerly *Donovania granulomatis*); it is seen in Giemsa-stained sections as a dark-staining, encapsulated, intracellular rod-shaped inclusion in macrophages, the so-called **Donovan body.** The disease is endemic in tropical areas such as New Guinea, southern India, and southern Africa.

Treatment

Treat with **doxycycline** or **TMP-SMX.**

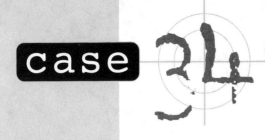

case

ID/CC A **60-year-old man** presents with **cough productive of mucopurulent sputum** together with mild fever and worsening breathlessness.

HPI He is a chronic smoker who has been diagnosed with **COPD.**

PE VS: fever. PE: in moderate respiratory distress; emphysematous chest with obliterated cardiac and liver dullness; **wheezing and crackles** heard over both lung fields.

Labs Organisms seen as small, pleomorphic gram-negative bacilli on Gram stain of sputum; **growth of organism on both factor X–hematin and factor V–nicotinamide nucleoside present in erythrocytes.**

case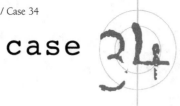

Haemophilus influenzae Infection in a COPD Patient

Differential

Bronchiectasis

Community-Acquired Pneumonia

α-Antitrypsin Deficiency

Lung Abscess

Tuberculosis

Legionnaire Disease

Discussion

Infections caused by nontypable, or unencapsulated, *Haemophilus influenzae* strains have been increasingly recognized in pediatric and adult populations. Nontypable *H. influenzae* strains are frequent respiratory tract colonizers in patients with COPD and commonly exacerbate chronic bronchitis in these patients; nontypable strains are also the most common cause of acute otitis media in children.

Treatment

Amoxicillin/ampicillin therapy; alternatively, TMP-SMX, azithromycin, or cefuroxime.

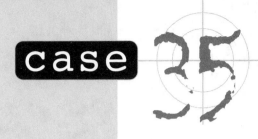

case 35

ID/CC A 20-year-old man presents with an extensive **purpuric skin rash, oliguria,** and marked weakness; he also complains of **bloody diarrhea** of 1 week's duration.

HPI The patient ate **a hamburger** at a fast-food restaurant 2 to 3 **days prior to the onset** of his diarrhea. He has no associated fever.

PE VS: no fever. PE: dehydration; pallor; extensive purpuric skin rash.

Labs Stool examination reveals the presence of RBCs but **no inflammatory cells** or parasites; culture isolates sorbitol-negative *Escherichia coli*; serotyping studies and effect on HeLa cell culture reveal presence of **enterohemorrhagic** *E. coli* (EHEC) **serotype O157: H7;** elevated BUN and creatinine. CBC/PBS: **microangiopathic anemia** and thrombocytopenia. PT, PTT normal.

Imaging Sigmoidoscopy: moderately hyperemic mucosa with no evidence of any ulceration.

Micro Pathology Pathology localized to the kidney, where hyaline **thrombi** were seen **in afferent arterioles** and glomerular capillaries.

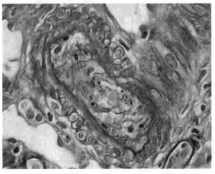

Figure 35-1. Renal arteriolar obliteration by a fibrin thrombus.

case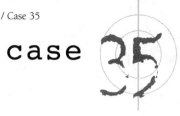

Hemolytic-Uremic Syndrome (HUS)

Differential

Thrombotic Thrombocytopenic Purpura (TTP)

Henoch-Schönlein Purpura

Disseminated Intravascular Coagulation (DIC)

Vasculitis

Acute Post-Streptococcal Glomerulonephritis

Discussion

Hemorrhagic colitis associated with a Shigalike toxin producing **EHEC O157:H7** is characterized by grossly bloody diarrhea with remarkably little fever or inflammatory exudate in stool; a significant number of patients develop potentially fatal HUS. EHEC infections can be largely **prevented through adequate cooking of beef,** especially hamburgers.

Treatment

Dialysis and blood transfusion for management of HUS; fluid and electrolyte maintenance; antimicrobial therapy. Most patients who develop HUS as a complication of E. *coli* hemorrhagic colitis die as a result of hemorrhagic complications.

case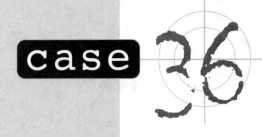

ID/CC A **3-year-old** White boy presents with golden-yellow, crusted lesions around his mouth and behind his ears.

HPI He has a history of intermittent low-grade fever, frequent "nose picking," and purulent discharge from his lesions. He has no history of hematuria (due to increased risk of poststreptococcal glomerulonephritis).

PE Characteristic **honey-colored crusted lesions** seen at **angle of mouth,** around nasal orifices, and behind ears.

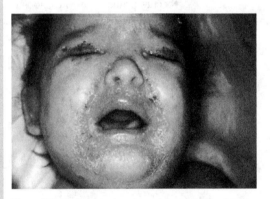

Figure 36-1. Honey-colored crusts on mouth and nose.

Labs **Gram-positive cocci in chains** (STREPTOCOCCI) in addition to pus cells on Gram stain of discharge; β-hemolytic streptococci (group A streptococci) on blood agar culture; ASO titer negative.

Gross Pathology Erythematous lesions surrounding natural orifices with whitish or yellowish purulent exudate and crust formation.

Micro Pathology Inflammatory infiltrate of PMNs with varying degrees of necrosis.

case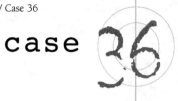

Impetigo

Differential

Erythema Multiforme

Herpes Simplex

Pediculosis

Staphylococcal Infection

Tinea Infection

Discussion

Impetigo is a highly communicable infectious disease that is most often caused by group A streptococci, occurs primarily in preschoolers, and may predispose to glomerulonephritis. It occurs most commonly on the face (periorbital area), hands, and arms. *Staphylococcus aureus* may coexist or cause bullous impetigo; group B streptococcal impetigo may be seen in newborns.

Treatment

Cephalosporin, penicillin, or erythromycin if allergic.

case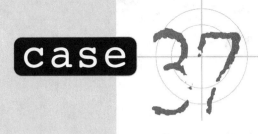

ID/CC A 30-year-old woman presents with **fever, chills,** malaise, headaches, and **myalgias.**

HPI She was diagnosed as suffering from **secondary syphilis** with an extensive nonpruritic **skin rash, condylomata lata,** and **mucous patches** in the mouth, for which she received a dose of intramuscular **penicillin 6 hours ago.**

PE VS: **fever;** tachycardia; mild hypotension.

Micro Swab of lesions demonstrates **spiral-shaped organisms** by **dark-field microscopy.**

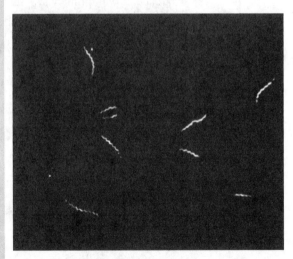

Figure 37-1. Dark-field microscopic examination depicts spiral organisms.

case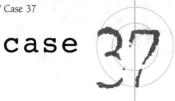

Jarisch-Herxheimer Reaction

Differential

Sepsis

Drug Reaction

Malaria

Mazzotti Reaction

Discussion

The Jarisch-Herxheimer reaction consists of fever, chills, mild hypotension, headache, and an increase in the intensity of mucocutaneous lesions **2 hours after** initiating **treatment of syphilis with penicillin** or another effective antibiotic; symptoms usually **subside in 12 to 24 hours.** The reaction occurs in 50% of patients with primary syphilis and in 90% of those with secondary syphilis. The Jarisch-Herxheimer reaction **also occurs after treatment of other spirochetal diseases** (e.g., louse-borne relapsing fever caused by *Borrelia recurrentis*). It has been suggested that the release of treponemal lipopolysaccharides might produce this symptom complex.

Treatment

No specific treatment; symptoms subside in 24 hours.

case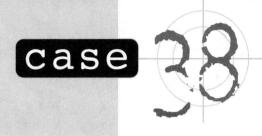

ID/CC	A 40-year-old smoker complains of acute-onset **high fever,** chills, a **nonproductive cough,** tachypnea, and **pleuritic chest pain.**
HPI	He also says that a number of **similar cases** have been reported in his workplace in recent months. The patient admits to significant alcohol and tobacco consumption and uses a **humidifier** at night.
PE	VS: fever; dyspnea. PE: rales present bilaterally on auscultation.
Labs	Sputum exam with Gram stain reveals no pathogenic organisms. CBC: neutrophilic leukocytosis. Urine ELISA is positive for **Legionella antigen;** sputum culture isolates *Legionella;* cold agglutinins absent; indirect fluorescent antibody technique reveals stable titer of >1:256 (considered diagnostic); **direct immunofluorescent** staining of sputum confirms presence of *Legionella.*
Imaging	CXR, PA: bilateral diffuse, patchy infiltrates and **ill-defined nodules.**
Gross Pathology	Nodular areas of consolidation that may progress to involvement of one or more lobes of the lung.
Micro Pathology	Alveolar exudate with PMNs, macrophages, and fibrin; in more severe cases, destruction of alveolar septa.

case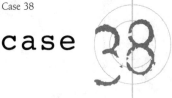

Legionella Pneumonia

Differential

Congestive Heart Failure
Costochondritis
Community-Acquired Pneumonia
Viral Pneumonia
Pleural Effusion
Q Fever

Discussion

Legionnaire's disease is caused by *Legionella pneumophila*, a filamentous, flagellated, aerobic gram-negative, motile bacillus, and is more common in immunocompromised patients. Epidemiologic studies have established **drinking water** and **air conditioners** as the sources of outbreaks.

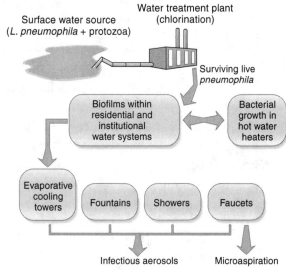

Figure 38-1. Sources of *Legionella* infection in humans.

Breakout Point

Pontiac Fever
A less severe form of infection caused by *Legionella*, characterized by fevers, chills, myalgia, malaise, and headache.

Treatment

Fluoroquinolone or macrolide therapy.

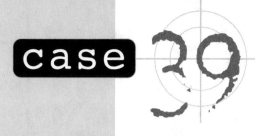

ID/CC A 30-year-old man from **India** presents with slowly progressive **hypopigmented skin patches and nodules** together with a peculiar **deformity of the nose.**

HPI The patient has a history of **nasal stuffiness** and bloody nasal discharge; he also complains of **loss of libido.**

PE **Leonine facies** (thickened facial and forehead skin); loss of eyebrows and eyelashes (MADAROSIS); scleral nodules; **depressed nasal bridge** ("SADDLE-NOSE" DEFORMITY); gynecomastia; **testicular atrophy;** numerous **symmetrical, hypopigmented macules with vague edges** and erythematous, smooth, shiny surfaces; skin plaques and nodules; **partial loss of pinprick and temperature sensation** (HYPOESTHESIA); no anhidrotic changes; symmetrically **enlarged ulnar and common peroneal nerves.**

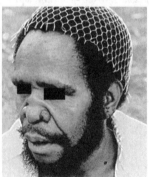

Figure 39-1. Leonine facies.

Labs CBC: mild anemia. ESR elevated; slit skin smears reveal **numerous acid-fast bacilli** on modified ZN staining.

Micro Pathology Dermis massively and diffusely infiltrated with **foamy histiocytes with bacilli and globi** (masses of acid-fast bacilli) containing Virchow giant cells; bacilli found only rarely in epidermis and in subepidermal **"clear zone";** epidermis thinned out with flattening of rete ridges.

case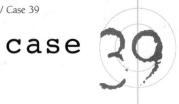

Leprosy—Lepromatous

Differential

Bell Palsy

Diabetic Neuropathy

Neurofibromatosis

Leishmaniasis

Eczema

Sarcoidosis

Discussion

The discovery of one or more of the following is pathognomonic of leprosy: (1) **anesthetic skin lesions** (found in all tuberculoid and many lepromatous cases); (2) **thickening of one or more nerves** (found in many lepromatous and some tuberculoid cases); and (3) the presence of **acid-fast bacilli in skin smears** (found in all lepromatous and some tuberculoid cases). *Mycobacterium leprae* has not been cultured in vitro thus far. Frequent complications include hand crippling (secondary to nerve damage) and blindness. It is currently believed that in most instances, the mode of transmission is via person-to-person contact.

Treatment

Multidrug therapy with **rifampicin, dapsone, and clofazimine.**

case 40

ID/CC A 26-year-old man from India presents with a **hypopigmented, anesthetic skin patch** over the left side of his face.

HPI He also complains of an occasional "electric current"-like sensation radiating from his left elbow to his hand.

PE Dry, hypopigmented, anesthetic patch over the left cheek; left **ulnar nerve enlarged and palpable;** eye, ear, nose, and throat exam normal; testes normal (versus signs that are often demonstrable in lepromatous leprosy).

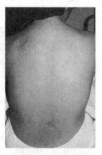

Figure 40-1. Multiple plaques, nodules, and hypopigmented patches.

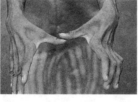

Figure 40-2. Muscular atrophy and claw hand deformity secondary to bilateral ulnar nerve palsy.

Labs Glucose-6-phosphate dehydrogenase (G6PD) levels within normal range (done to prevent dapsone-associated hemolysis); slit skin smears reveal few **acid-fast bacilli;** skin biopsy from patch diagnostic of tuberculoid leprosy.

Gross Pathology **Single or small number of lesions** with macular or raised edges.

Micro Pathology Skin biopsy reveals many well-formed epithelioid granulomas with very **few** acid-fast bacilli.

case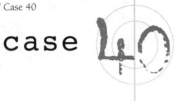

Leprosy—Tuberculoid

Differential

Systemic Lupus Erythematosus
Kaposi Sarcoma
Neurofibromatosis
Leishmaniasis
Syphilis
Mycobacterium marinum Infection

Discussion

Caused by *Mycobacterium leprae,* an acid-fast bacillus. The organism has two unique properties: it is thermolabile, growing best at 27°C to 30°C, and it divides very slowly; generation time is 12 to 14 days. Consequently, leprosy in humans typically evolves very slowly. Tuberculoid leprosy predominantly affects the skin with limited nerve involvement (most commonly ulnar and peroneal); **lepromatous leprosy** has diffuse involvement of the skin, eyes, nerves, and upper airway with disfigurement of the hands and face **(leonine facies).**

Treatment

Chemotherapy with rifampin and dapsone.

case

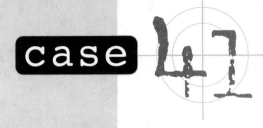

ID/CC	A 35-year-old British **dairy farmer** complains of a high remittent **fever** with chills, severe muscle aches, **decreased urine output**, and **dark-colored urine** for the past 2 days.
HPI	He also complains of an extensive skin rash and nasal bleeding (EPISTAXIS). A careful history reveals that the area in which he works is infested with rodents.
PE	VS: **fever**; tachycardia; hypotension. PE: **icterus**; extensive hemorrhagic maculopapular skin eruption; **conjunctival suffusion**; lymphadenopathy.
Labs	CBC: leukocytosis with neutrophilia; thrombocytopenia. Mild **hyperbilirubinemia,** predominantly conjugated; **increased alkaline phosphatase; elevated BUN and creatinine.** UA: proteinuria, **casts,** and RBCs.
Imaging	CXR: patchy alveolar infiltrates consistent with alveolar hemorrhage.
Gross Pathology	Severe infection damages both the **liver and kidneys.**
Micro Pathology	Liver biopsy shows focal centrilobular necrosis with focal lymphocytic infiltration and disorganization of liver cell plates together with proliferation of Kupffer cells with cholestasis; kidney biopsy reveals mesangial proliferation with PMN infiltration.

case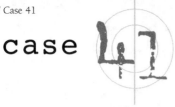

Leptospirosis (Weil Disease)

Differential

Hepatitis
Kawasaki Disease
Yellow Fever
Brucellosis
Pancreatitis
Hemorrhagic Fever

Discussion

Weil disease, a severe form of leptospirosis caused by *Leptospira interrogans* complex, is characterized by fever, jaundice, cutaneous and visceral hemorrhages, anemia, azotemia, and altered consciousness; major vectors to humans are rodents. Transmission occurs through direct contact with the blood, tissue, or urine of infected animals. Person-to-person transmission is highly unlikely. Preventive measures include limiting the rodent population and vaccinating animals.

Treatment

IV penicillin; doxycycline for uncomplicated infections; supportive therapy for multiorgan failure.

case 42

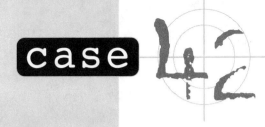

ID/CC   A **neonate died** shortly after birth.

HPI   Review of the medical record reveals history of **refusal to feed,** an extensive **maculopapular skin rash** on his legs and trunk, **respiratory distress,** diarrhea, and seizures shortly after birth.

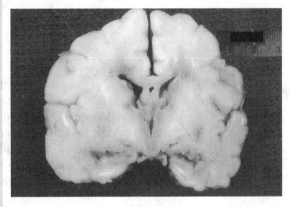

Figure 42-1. Swollen brain parenchyma with opaque meninges.

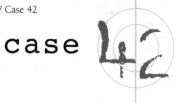

Listeria Meningitis in the Newborn

Differential

Bacteremia

Neonatal Sepsis

Pneumonia

Urinary Tract Infection

Herpes Meningitis

TORCH Group (**T**oxoplasmosis, **O**ther infections, **R**ubella, **C**ytomegalovirus infection, and **H**erpes simplex) Infection

Discussion

Neonatal listeriosis may occur early or late in neonatal life. Infants may be acutely ill at birth and may die within hours as a result of disseminated listeriosis, which is also called **granulomatosis infantiseptica**. This condition is characterized by **hepatosplenomegaly, thrombocytopenia,** generalized **skin papules,** whitish pharyngeal patches, and **pneumonia.** Commonly, a stained smear of meconium will reveal **gram-positive bacilli,** suggesting the diagnosis.

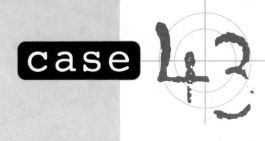

ID/CC A **2-week-old** girl is brought to the emergency room because of **high fever and convulsions.**

HPI She also has an **extensive skin rash** on her legs and trunk.

PE VS: fever. PE: generalized hypotonia; **extensive maculopapular skin rash; nuchal rigidity; involuntary flexion of hips when flexing neck** (BRUDZINSKI SIGN).

Labs CBC: neutrophilic leukocytosis. LP: elevated CSF cell count (750 cells/mL), mostly **neutrophils;** elevated CSF protein; low CSF sugar. Gram-positive, facultative, intracellular, nonsporulating motile bacilli on Gram stain and culture.

Gross Pathology Purulent meningitis.

Micro Pathology Bacillus provokes both acute suppurative reaction with neutrophilic infiltration and chronic granuloma formation with focal necrosis.

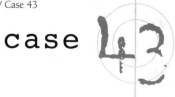

case

Listeriosis

Differential

Bacteremia
Neonatal Sepsis
Pneumonia
Urinary Tract Infection
Herpes Meningitis
TORCH Group (**T**oxoplasmosis, **O**ther infections, **R**ubella, **C**ytomegalovirus infection, and **H**erpes simplex) Infection.

Discussion

Listeriosis is caused by **Listeria monocytogenes.** Bacterial infection may occur early (acquired **in utero**) or later (drinking **contaminated milk**) in neonatal life. May be rapidly fatal if disseminated. Also occurs in adults immunocompromised by disease (e.g., renal disease or HIV). *Escherichia coli* and group B streptococci are two other common causes of neonatal meningitis.

■ **TABLE 43-1 SERIOUS BACTERIAL INFECTIONS IN INFANTS: COMMON ORGANISMS**

Bacteremia-meningitis	Gastroenteritis
<30 days	*Salmonella* species
Group B streptococci	*Shigella* species
Escherichia coli	*Yersinia enterolytica*
Listeria monocytogenes	*Campylobacter*
>30 days	Urinary tract infection
Group B streptococci	*E. coli*
E. coli	*Klebsiella pneumoniae*
Salmonella species	Group B streptococci
Streptococcus pneumoniae	Enterococcus
Haemophilus influenzae type b	Osteomyelitis
Neisseria meningitidis	Group B streptococci
	E. coli
	Staphylococcus aureus

Breakout Point

Listeria are facultative intracellular organisms that can spread from cell to cell by the induction of actin polymerization, which propels the organism from cell to cell (actin rocket). This cell-to-cell transmission allows the infection to spread while evading humoral immunity.

Treatment

IV antibiotics (high-dose ampicillin).

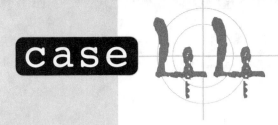

case

ID/CC A 12-year-old boy presents with **fatigue, fever,** headache, **fleeting joint pain,** and a **reddish rash** on his trunk and left leg of 1 week's duration.

HPI The patient is a native of **Connecticut** and attended a summer camp in the state's national park 2 weeks ago. He recalls having noticed a **tick bite** on his leg about 2 weeks ago.

PE VS: fever. PE: red macule on site of bite that has grown circumferentially; **active border and central clearing** (ERYTHEMA CHRONICUM MIGRANS); femoral lymphadenopathy; mild neck stiffness; normal CNS exam.

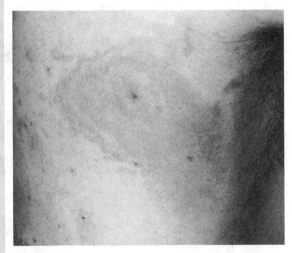

Figure 44-1. Primary erythema chronicum migrans lesion.

Labs ECG: normal. LP: lymphocytic pleocytosis; increased proteins.

Gross Pathology Erythema chronicum migrans (ECM) must be a minimum of 5 cm in diameter for the diagnosis to be made; the center may desquamate, ulcerate, or necrose; satellite lesions sometimes are seen; may spontaneously disappear with time.

87

case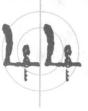

Lyme Disease

Differential

Fibromyalgia
Gonococcal Arthritis
Gout
Rheumatoid Arthritis
Systemic Lupus Erythematosus
Psoriatic Arthritis

Discussion

The most common disease transmitted by vectors in the United States, Lyme disease is caused by *Borrelia burgdorferi*, a spirochete, and is transmitted through *Ixodes* species tick bites. Ticks acquire *B. burgdorferi* from deer mice, which are the natural reservoir. There are three recognized stages: stage 1 consists of ECM and constitutional symptoms; stage 2, cardiac or neurologic involvement; and stage 3, persistent migratory arthritis, synovitis, and **atrophic patches on the distal extremities** (ACRODERMATITIS CHRONICUM ATROPHICANS).

■ TABLE 44-1 CLINICAL STAGES OF LYME DISEASE

Stage 1: Early infection
   Erythema migrans
   Flulike symptoms
   Regional adenopathy
Stage 2: Disseminated infection
   Multiple erythema migrans lesions
   Hepatitis, musculoskeletal complaints
   Acute neurologic disease
   Cranial nerve palsies, especially VII
   Meningitis
   Cardiac involvement
   Atrioventricular block
Stage 3: Late disease
   Arthritis
   Neurologic syndromes
   Encephalitis
   Radiculopathies
   Late skin involvement

Treatment

Doxycycline; amoxicillin; ceftriaxone.

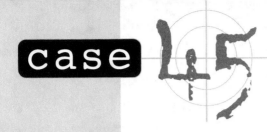

ID/CC A 50-year-old white man develops **sudden fever with chills,** pain in the back and extremities, and **neck stiffness;** he vomited six times and had a **convulsion** prior to admission.

HPI The patient is a **heavy smoker** and is **diabetic. Two weeks ago,** he had a **URI.** He is also very sensitive to light (PHOTOPHOBIA).

PE Markedly reduced mental status (OBTUNDED); petechial rash over trunk and abdomen; **nuchal and spinal rigidity; positive Kernig and Brudzinski signs;** no focal neurologic deficits.

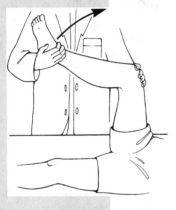

Figure 45-1. Kernig sign. With the patient lying on his or her back, flex one of the patient's legs at the hip and knee. If pain or resistance is elicited as the knee is straightened, this is a positive Kernig sign.

Labs LP: **elevated pressure; cloudy CSF; elevated protein; markedly decreased glucose; high cell count with mostly WBCs.** CSF Gram stain reveals **gram-positive diplococci.**

Imaging CT/MR, brain: **meningeal thickening** and enhancement.

Gross Pathology Pia-arachnoid congestion results from inflammatory infiltrate; a thin layer of pus forms and promotes adhesions while obstructing normal CSF flow (can cause hydrocephalus); brain is covered with purulent exudate, most heavily on the base.

case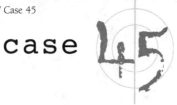

Meningitis—Bacterial (Adult)

Differential
CNS Vasculitis
Meningeal Carcinomatosis
Herpes Encephalitis
Sinusitis
Stroke
Brain Abscess
Viral Meningitis

Discussion
Bacterial meningitis is a pyogenic infection of the CNS that requires prompt treatment. *Streptococcus pneumoniae* is the most common cause of adult meningitis.

■ TABLE 45-1 CSF FINDINGS IN MENINGITIS AND OTHER CONDITIONS

Diagnosis	RBCs	Mono	PMNs	CSF Pressure (mm Hg)	Glucose (mg/dL)	Protein (mg/dL)
Normal CSF	0	<5	0	<200	40–75	15–55
Bacterial	N	+	+ + +	+	<40	>55
Aseptic meningitis	N	+ +	+	+	N	+
Amebic, protozoan, fungal, tubercular	N	+ + +	+	+	<40	+
Spirochete, viral	N, +	+ +[a]	+	+	N	+
Subarachnoid hemorrhage	+ + +	+	+	+ +	N	+ +
CNS neoplasm	N	N	N	+ +	N	+ +

[a]A PMN reaction can be seen in this early CNS infection. This usually converts within a short time to a mononuclear majority.

+, + +, + + +, increased; CNS, central nervous system; CSF, cerebrospinal fluid; Mono, mononuclear leukocytes; N, normal; PMN, polymorphonuclear leukocytes; RBCs, red blood cells.

Breakout Point

Common Causes of Meningitis in Adult Populations:
Ages 6 years to 60 years—Enterovirus Military recruits and dormitory residents—Meningococci Elderly (>60 years old)—Pneumococci

Treatment
Early empiric high-dose IV antibiotics; cefotaxime; vancomycin; high-dose steroids.

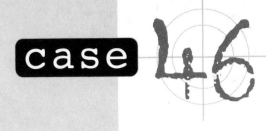

case 46

ID/CC A **4-year-old** girl presents with a 1-week history of **fever**, severe **headache, irritability**, and **malaise**; 2 days ago she developed **neck stiffness**, and her parents report **projectile vomiting** over the past 24 hours.

HPI The child is also very sensitive to light (PHOTOPHOBIA). She is fully immunized and has no history of ear, nose, and throat infection, skin rashes, dog bites, or foreign travel.

PE VS: fever. PE: irritability; resistance to being touched or moved; minimal papilledema of fundus; no focal neurologic signs; no cranial nerve deficits; positive **Kernig** and **Brudzinski** signs.

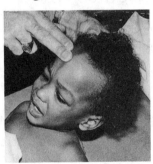

Figure 46-1. Nuchal rigidity with resisting flexion of the neck.

Labs CBC: **neutrophilic leukocytosis.** LP: increased pressure; **cloudy CSF; neutrophilic pleocytosis; decreased glucose; increased protein; gram-negative coccobacilli.** Negative ZN and India ink staining; normal serum electrolytes.

Imaging CT/MR, brain: **meningeal thickening** and enhancement.

Gross Pathology Abundant accumulation of purulent exudate between pia mater and arachnoid; meningeal thickening; cloudy to frankly purulent CSF.

Micro Pathology Intense neutrophilic infiltrate.

91

case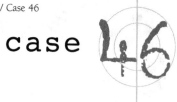

Meningitis—Bacterial (Pediatric)

Differential
Brain Abscess
Pseudotumor Cerebri
Brain Tumor
CNS Leukemia
Lead Encephalopathy
Viral Meningitis

Discussion
A pyogenic infection of the nervous system primarily affecting the meninges, bacterial meningitis is most commonly caused by pneumococcus (*Streptococcus pneumoniae*, associated with sickle cell anemia), meningococcus (*Neisseria meningitidis*, associated with a petechial skin rash), and *Haemophilus influenzae* (most commonly in children). It is less commonly caused by enterobacteria, *Streptococcus* species, *Staphylococcus* species (due to dental infection), and anaerobic organisms (due to trauma).

Breakout Point

Common Causes of Meningitis in Children
Ages 0–6 months: Group B streptococci, *Escherichia coli, Listeria*
Ages 6 months–6 years: *H. influenzae* type b (decreasing), *S. pneumoniae*, Enterovirus

Treatment
IV antibiotics (ampicillin, cefotaxime); consider steroids.

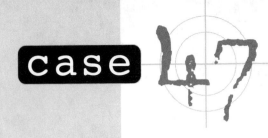

ID/CC	A **6-year-old boy** being treated for **primary pulmonary tuberculosis** presents with **diplopia**, increasing drowsiness, irritability, and unexplained, recurrent **vomiting**.
HPI	The child has had a low-grade fever, loss of appetite, and a persistent headache over the past few weeks.
PE	VS: fever. PE: stuporous; signs of meningeal irritation noted (**neck rigidity, Kernig sign, Brudzinski sign**); **CN III and IV palsy** on the right side; funduscopy reveals **papilledema**.

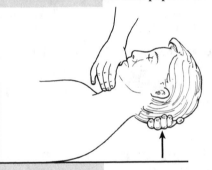

Figure 47-1. Brudzinski sign. With the patient lying on his or her back, place your hand behind the patient's neck and flex the neck toward the sternum. In a patient with meningeal irritation there is neck pain, neck stiffness, and flexion of the hips and knees.

Labs	LP (guarded): CSF under **increased pressure** and **turbid**; on standing, a **"cobweb" coagulum** formed at the center of the tube; CSF studies reveal **lymphocytic pleocytosis**, greatly **elevated protein**, and **low sugar**; ZN staining of CSF coagulum reveals presence of **acid-fast bacilli**.
Imaging	CT: suggests **basal exudates, inflammatory granulomas**, and a **communicating hydrocephalus**; striking meningeal enhancement is noted in post-contrast studies.
Micro Pathology	Subarachnoid space contains gelatinous exudate of chronic inflammatory cells, obliterating cisterns, and encasing cranial nerves; well-formed **granulomas** occasionally seen, most often at the base of the brain; arteries running through subarachnoid space show "obliterative endarteritis."

case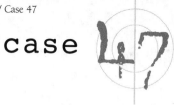

Meningitis—Tubercular

Differential

Brain Abscess
Fungal Meningitis
Viral Meningitis
CNS Vasculitis
Sarcoidosis

Discussion

Tuberculous infection reaches the meninges through the hematogenous route, resulting in a clinically sub-acute form of meningitis; it is often complicated by cranial nerve palsies, a communicating hydrocephalus, decerebrate posturing, convulsions, coma, and death.

Treatment

Antituberculous therapy with rifampin, isoniazid, ethambutol, and pyrazinamide; steroids; ventriculoperitoneal shunt to relieve hydrocephalus.

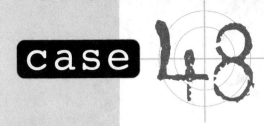

case 48

ID/CC A 12-year-old white boy is brought to the emergency room because of sudden **fever** with **chills, severe headache,** pain in the extremities and back, **stiff neck,** and generalized rash; he also **fainted** while in school.

HPI He had been well until admission, with no relevant history. In the emergency room, he **vomits bright red blood** twice.

PE VS: tachycardia; hypotension (BP 70/50 mm Hg). PE: altered sensorium; pallor; moist, cold skin; nuchal rigidity and positive Kernig's sign; **purpuric rash** all over body; minimal papilledema on funduscopic exam; no focal neurologic signs.

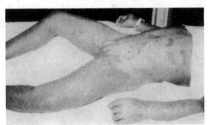

Figure 48-1. Widespread purpuric rash in patient.

Labs **Hypoglycemia.** Lytes: **hyponatremia; hyperkalemia.** CBC/PBS: thrombocytopenia; **neutrophilic leukocytosis.** LP: **CSF** cloudy and under increased pressure; increased proteins; low sugar. **Gram-negative diplococci** seen **within and outside WBCs** on Gram stain; negative India ink and ZN stain.

Imaging CT, head: normal. CT, abdomen: bilateral adrenal hemorrhage.

Gross Pathology **Bilateral adrenal hemorrhagic necrosis;** skin necrosis; pyogenic meningitis.

Micro Pathology Meningeal hyperemia with abundant purulent exudate; diplococcus-containing PMNs; acute hemorrhagic necrosis of adrenal glands.

case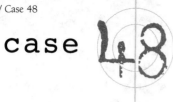

Meningococcemia

Differential

Gonococcal Infection

Rocky Mountain Spotted Fever

Thrombotic Thrombocytopenic Purpura

Hemorrhagic Fever

Disseminated Intravascular Coagulation

Discussion

Meningococcemia is a **fulminant disease** caused by several groups of *Neisseria meningitidis;* the cause of death is adrenal necrosis with vascular collapse. A meningococcal vaccine is available. Also known as **Waterhouse–Friderichsen syndrome.**

Treatment

Steroid replacement; IV fluids; dopamine; IV penicillin or ceftriaxone; prophylactic rifampin or ciprofloxacin for close contacts.

Breakout Point

> A meningococcal polysaccharide vaccine is available and protects against the most common serotypes, including: A, C, Y, and W135.

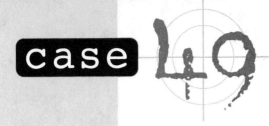

ID/CC A 20-year-old college student presents with a **productive cough**, headache, **malaise**, runny nose, and **fever.**

HPI He has a history of sore throat preceding the onset of the **cough, which initially was nonproductive.**

PE VS: fever. PE: mild respiratory distress; auscultation reveals fine to medium rales over the left middle lobe.

Labs Gram stain of sputum negative; routine cultures of both blood and sputum negative. CBC: **leukocyte count normal.** Fourfold rise in complement fixation titer in paired sera; **cold agglutinin titer** >1:128.

Imaging CXR: patchy alveolar infiltrates involving the left middle lobe; appears worse than the clinical picture.

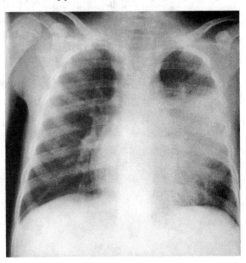

Figure 49-1. Left middle lobe infiltrate.

Gross Pathology Unilateral middle lobe pneumonia with firm, red pulmonary parenchyma in affected areas.

Micro Pathology Bronchial mucosa congested and edematous; inflammatory response consists of perivascular lymphocytes initially and PMNs later in infection.

case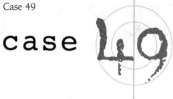

Mycoplasma Pneumonia

Differential

Bacterial Pneumonia

Viral Pneumonia

Chlamydia Pneumonia

Psittacosis

Q Fever

Discussion

Mycoplasma pneumoniae is the **most common cause of primary atypical pneumonia.** Transmission is by droplet spread; rapidly infects those living in close quarters.

Breakout Point

> ***Mycoplasma pneumoniae*** infection is associated with the development of cold **agglutinins** (usually IgM antibodies targeted against red blood cell antigens) with the subsequent development of hemolysis **(autoimmune hemolytic anemia).**

Treatment

Erythromycin. Organism lacks a cell wall and thus penicillins and cephalosporins are ineffective.

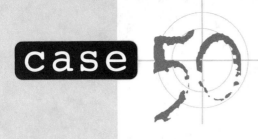

case 50

ID/CC	A 14-year-old **malnourished boy** died soon after hospitalization due to an **extensive small bowel rupture and shock.**
HPI	He had presented to the emergency room with **massive bloody diarrhea.** His history at admission revealed the presence of abdominal pain, fever, and diarrhea of a few days' duration; his symptoms had developed **after he ate leftover meat** at a fast-food restaurant.
PE	He was dehydrated, pale, and hypotensive at the time of admission and developed signs of peritonitis and shock shortly before his death.
Labs	Culture and exam of necrotizing intestinal lesions isolated *Clostridium perfringens* **type C** producing beta toxin.
Gross Pathology	Autopsy revealed a ruptured small intestine, mucosal ulcerations, and **gas production (pneumatosis)** in the wall.

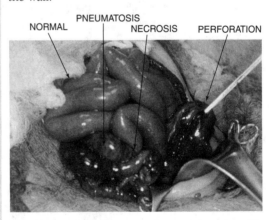

Figure 50-1. Extensive areas of necrotic intestine with characteristic pneumatosis can be seen adjacent to grossly normal bowel.

Micro Pathology	Microscopic exam revealed necrosis and acute inflammation in the ileum.

case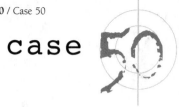

Necrotizing Enterocolitis

Differential

Sepsis

Intestinal Malrotation

Intestinal Volvulus

Omphalitis

Ruptured Megacolon

Discussion

Necrotizing enterocolitis is a condition affecting poorly nourished persons who suddenly feast on meat **(Pigbel)**. It is associated with *Clostridium perfringens* type C and **beta enterotoxin**; beta toxin paralyzes the villi and causes friability and necrosis of the bowel wall. Immunization of children in New Guinea with beta-toxoid vaccine has dramatically decreased the incidence of the disease.

Treatment

Patient died despite aggressive fluid and electrolyte replacement, bowel decompression, and antibiotic therapy (penicillin, clindamycin, or doxycycline); surgery had been planned in view of rupture of the small bowel.

case 51

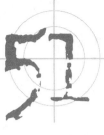

ID/CC A 50-year-old diabetic man presents with **fever, pain, and a necrotizing swelling** over his left arm.

HPI His symptoms began about a week ago with redness and swelling of the left arm followed by bronze discoloration of the skin and the appearance of hemorrhagic bullae.

PE Extensive cutaneous **gangrene** observed over the left arm with many ruptured bullae; black necrotic eschar with surrounding erythema resembles a third-degree burn.

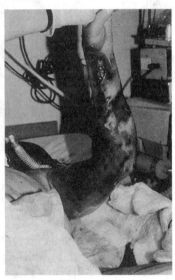

Figure 51-1. Characteristic rapidly evolving necrotic lesions of the extremity.

Labs Swab staining reveals the presence of chains of grampositive cocci; culture isolated β-**hemolytic group A streptococci** (*Streptococcus pyogenes*).

Micro Pathology Biopsy specimen reveals areas of necrosis in dermis and subcutaneous fat, infiltration with PMNs, and vasculitis and thrombosis in vessels in the superficial fascia.

case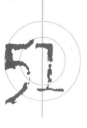

Necrotizing Fasciitis

Differential

Cellulitis
Gas Gangrene
Scalded Skin Syndrome
Chemical Burn
Burn
Nodular Vasculitis
Deep Vein Thrombosis

Discussion

Streptococcal gangrene is a group A streptococcal cellulitis that rapidly progresses to gangrene of the subcutaneous tissue and necrosis of the overlying skin; the disease process usually involves an extremity. Necrotizing fasciitis is also recognized as a polymicrobial infection that is caused by aerobes and anaerobes ("SYNERGISTIC NECROTIZING CELLULITIS"). Infection spreads quickly through various fascial planes, the venous system, and lymphatics. Predisposing etiologies include surgery, trauma, and diabetes.

Breakout Point

> β-Hemolytic group A streptococcal strains capable of causing necrotizing fasciitis are often called **"flesh-eating bacteria."**

Treatment

Treatment includes rapid **surgical excision of necrotic tissue** in combination with appropriate **antibiotics**; **penicillin G** is the drug of choice for streptococcal infection.

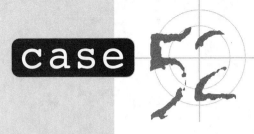

case 52

ID/CC A 7-year-old boy who has been hospitalized for treatment of **acute lymphocytic leukemia** complains of **copious watery diarrhea**, right lower quadrant **abdominal pain**, and **fever**.

HPI He was diagnosed as **neutropenic** (due to aggressive cytotoxic chemotherapy) a few days ago.

PE VS: fever; tachycardia; tachypnea. PE: pallor; sternal tenderness; axillary lymphadenopathy; hepatosplenomegaly; abdominal distention; moderate dehydration.

Labs CBC: severe **neutropenia**; anemia; thrombocytopenia. PBS and bone marrow studies suggest he is in remission; blood culture grows ***Clostridium septicum.***

Imaging CT, abdomen: **thickening of cecal wall.**

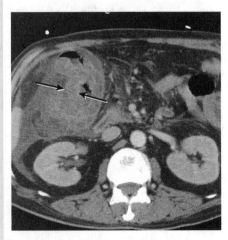

Figure 52-1. There is concentric mural thickening in the hepatic flexure. The wall thickening is severe (*arrows*).

Gross Pathology Mucosal ulcers and inflammation in the **ileocecal region** of the small intestine.

103

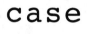 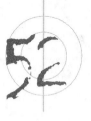

Neutropenic Enterocolitis

Differential
Crohn Disease
Appendicitis
Diverticulitis
Ulcerative Colitis
CMV Colitis
Acute Megacolon
Ogilvie Syndrome

Discussion
Neutropenic enterocolitis is a fulminant form of necrotizing enteritis that occurs in neutropenic patients; neutropenia is often related to cyclic neutropenia, leukemia, aplastic anemia, or chemotherapy. In postmortem exams of patients who have died of leukemia, infections of the cecal area (TYPHLITIS) are frequently found; *Clostridium septicum* is the most common organism isolated from the blood of such patients.

Treatment
Aggressive **supportive measures**; surgical intervention; appropriate **antibiotics** (penicillin G, ampicillin, or clindamycin).

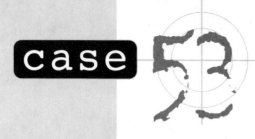

ID/CC   A 45-year-old white man undergoing **chemotherapy** for Hodgkin lymphoma is brought to the emergency room by his wife because of shortness of breath and cyanosis.

HPI   For the past **3 months**, he has been complaining of intermittent weakness, fever with chills, and foul-smelling, thick **greenish sputum**.

PE   VS: fever (38°C); tachypnea; tachycardia. PE: pallor; mild cyanosis; localized dullness with bronchial breathing; diminished breath sounds over the left lower lobe.

Labs   CBC: leukocytosis with neutrophilia; anemia. Sputum culture reveals **gram-positive, filamentous, partially acid-fast** staining bacteria.

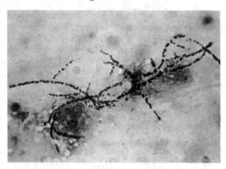

Figure 53-1. Gram stain of organisms from the sputum of a patient. The organisms appear as a beaded, gram-positive, branching tangle adjacent to three necrotic white cells.

Imaging   CXR: nodular infiltrate in left lower lobe with air-fluid level (abscess) and left pleural effusion.

Gross Pathology   Lung lesions or disseminated lesions (brain, liver, kidney, subcutaneous tissue) consist of necrotic centers within regions of consolidation and abscess formation resembling pyogenic pneumonia.

Micro Pathology   Consolidation of alveoli with pus formation (exudate of PMNs and fibrin) and surrounding granulomatous reaction.

105

case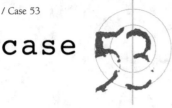

Nocardiosis

Differential

Actinomycosis

Aspergillosis

Histoplasmosis

Lung Abscess

Mycobacterium avium-intracellulare

Tuberculosis

Pneumocystis carinii Pneumonia

Discussion

A chronic bacterial infection seen in diabetics, leukemia and lymphoma patients, and **immunocompromised patients,** nocardiosis usually involves the lungs with possible dissemination to the brain, subcutaneous tissue, and other organs. It is caused by ***Nocardia asteroides,*** a branching, aerobic, gram-positive organism that is weakly acid fast and is sometimes confused with *Mycobacterium tuberculosis.*

Treatment

Six-month course of TMP-SMX; surgery.

case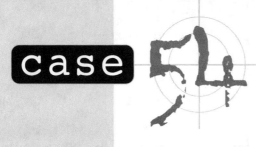

ID/CC   A 60-year-old man who was hospitalized following a stroke presents with a high-grade **fever with chills** and obtundation.

HPI   He had been **catheterized due to urinary incontinence and was receiving cephalosporin** for treatment of aspiration pneumonitis.

PE   VS: fever.

Labs   **Blood culture** grew colonies morphologically indistinguishable from streptococci and immunologically similar to members of group D streptococci, the enterococci are metabolically unique in their ability to resist heat, bile, and 6.5% sodium chloride; urine culture also isolated the same organisms.

case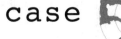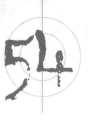

Nosocomial Enterococcal Infection

Differential

Sepsis

Pyelonephritis

Cystitis

Adrenal Insufficiency

Prostatitis

Discussion

Enterococci constitute a relatively common cause of UTIs, wound infections, and peritonitis and intra-abdominal abscesses; they have also become an increasingly prominent cause of **bacteremia,** which usually originates from a **focus in the urinary tract or abdomen.** The incidence of nosocomial bacteremias caused by these organisms is also increasing, particularly in patients who have received cephalosporins or other broad-spectrum antibiotics. All clinically significant isolates should be subjected to testing for β-**lactamase production,** high-level **aminoglycoside resistance,** and **vancomycin resistance** to determine if an alternative therapy is necessary. Infections caused by enterococci that produce β-lactamase are treated with an antimicrobial agent that combines a penicillin with a β-lactamase inhibitor; infections caused by strains that are highly resistant to aminoglycosides are treated with vancomycin.

Treatment

Ampicillin with gentamicin (vancomycin can be substituted for ampicillin in patients with penicillin allergies).

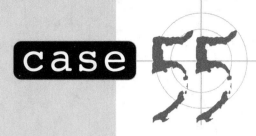

case 55

ID/CC   A 4-year-old white boy presents with fever, chills, malaise, **pain,** and **immobility of the right knee** of 1 week's duration.

HPI   Two weeks ago the child fell while playing, but no abnormality was found by the school nurse.

PE   Overlying skin **warm and red; swelling** of distal third of thigh and knee; **tenderness** on palpation.

Labs   CBC: leukocytosis. **Elevated ESR.** Gram stain and culture confirm diagnosis and isolate pathogen.

Imaging   XR, plain: early findings include soft tissue edema and thin line running parallel to diaphysis **(periosteal thickening);** later findings include bone erosion, sub-periosteal abscess with periostitis, and sequestrum formation (due to detached necrotic cortical bone); involucrum formation (laminated periosteal reaction). Isolated localized abscess (BRODIE'S ABSCESS); MR: marrow edema; abscess. **Indium-labeled WBC scan: hot spot.**

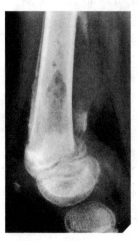

Figure 55-1. Radiograph shows widespread destruction of the cortical and medullary portions of the metaphysis and diaphysis of the distal femur, together with periosteal new bone formation.

Micro Pathology   Purulent exudate formation, usually metaphyseal, with ischemic necrosis of bone due to increased pressure of pus in rigid bone walls; vascular thrombosis.

109

case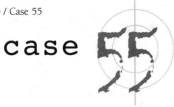

Osteomyelitis

Differential

Cellulitis

Gout

Septic Arthritis

Primary Bone Tumor

Gas Gangrene

Metastatic Tumor

Discussion

Osteomyelitis is an acute pyogenic bone infection that if left untreated, produces functional incapacity and deformities. The most common pathogen is **Staphylococcus aureus;** less frequently *Streptococcus* and enterobacteria are involved. In sickle cell anemia *Escherichia coli* and *Salmonella* species are seen; diabetics are at risk for *Pseudomonas* infection. Immunocompromised patients may show *Sporothrix schenckii* osteomyelitis; human bites, anaerobes; puncture wounds, *Pseudomonas aeruginosa*; and cat-bite wounds, *Pasteurella multocida*.

Treatment

IV antibiotics according to sensitivity; **surgical débridement.**

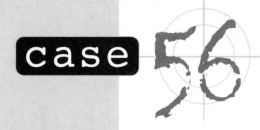

ID/CC A 20-year-old swimmer complains of severe **pain** and **itching** in the right ear that is associated with a slight amount of **yellowish** (PURULENT) **discharge.**

HPI He has no previous history of discharge from the ear and no history of associated deafness or tinnitus.

PE Red, swollen area seen in the right external auditory meatus that is partially obliterating the lumen; **movement of the tragus** is exquisitely **painful** (TRAGAL SIGN).

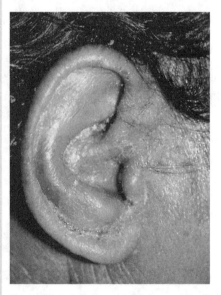

Figure 56-1. Infection extends beyond the limits of the canal to involve adjacent soft tissues. Erythema of the conchal skin and scaliness are secondary to profuse drainage.

Labs Gram stain of aural swab reveals presence of gram-negative rods; culture isolates *Pseudomonas aeruginosa.*

Gross Pathology Red, swollen area seen in cartilaginous part of external auditory meatus; when visualized, the tympanic membrane is erythematous and moves normally with pneumatic otoscopy (versus acute otitis media).

case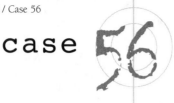

Otitis Externa

Differential

Otitis Media
Foreign Body in Ear
Chondritis
Intracranial Abscess
Cellulitis

Discussion

Otitis externa is most common in summer months and is thought to arise from a change in the milieu of the external auditory meatus by increased alkalization and excessive moisture; this leads to bacterial overgrowth, most commonly with gram-negative rods such as *Pseudomonas* (also causes malignant otitis externa) and *Proteus* or fungi such as *Aspergillus*.

Treatment

Eardrops (either a combination of polymyxin, neomycin, and hydrocortisone or ofloxacin); gentle removal of debris in ear.

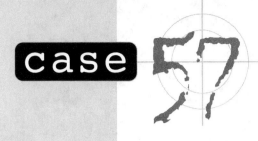

case 57

ID/CC An 18-month-old white girl presents with **irritability** together with a bilateral, profuse, and foul-smelling **ear discharge** of 2 months' duration.

HPI The patient had **recurrent URIs** last year, but her mother did not administer the complete course of antibiotics. The patient's mother has a history of feeding her child while lying down.

PE Bilateral greenish-white ear discharge; **perforated tympanic membranes** in anteroinferior quadrant of both ears; **diminished mobility of tympanic membrane** on pneumatic otoscopy.

Labs Gram-negative coccobacilli on Gram stain of discharge from tympanocentesis; *Haemophilus influenzae* seen on culture.

Gross Pathology Possible complications include **ingrowth of squamous epithelium on upper middle ear** (CHOLESTEATOMA) if long-standing; conductive hearing loss; mastoiditis; and brain abscess.

Micro Pathology Hyperemia and edema of inner ear and throat mucosa; hyperemia of tympanic membrane; deposition of cholesterol crystals in keratinized epidermoid cells in cholesteatoma.

case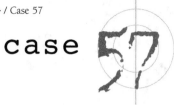

Otitis Media

Differential
Sinusitis
Foreign Body in Ear
Labyrinthitis
Mastoiditis
Peritonsillar Abscess
Otitis Externa

Discussion
Otitis media is the most common pediatric bacterial infection and is caused by *Escherichia coli, Staphylococcus aureus,* and *Klebsiella pneumoniae* in neonates; in older children it is usually caused by pneumococcus (*Streptococcus pneumoniae*), *H. influenzae, Moraxella catarrhalis,* and group A streptococci. Resistant strains are becoming increasingly common.

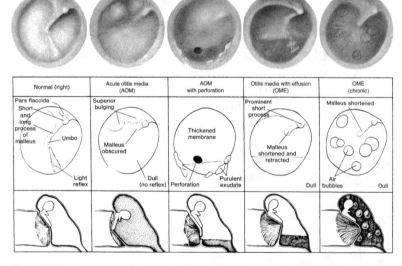

Figure 57-1. Appearance of the tympanic membrane in different types of otitis media.

Treatment
Keep ear dry; **amoxicillin-clavulanic acid;** surgical drainage for severe otalgia; myringoplasty.

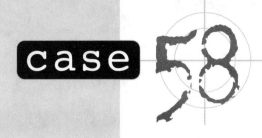

ID/CC A 9-year-old boy is admitted for an evaluation of a **suspected** underlying **immune deficiency.**

HPI He has been hospitalized and treated several times for **recurrent** life-threatening **septicemia due to *Streptococcus pneumoniae,* meningococcus,** and *Haemophilus influenzae.* Careful history reveals that a few years ago he underwent an emergency **splenectomy** following traumatic splenic rupture in a motor vehicle accident.

PE Left paramedian postsurgical scar seen on abdomen.

Labs Reduced IgM levels; **reduced antibody production when challenged with particulate antigens;** PBS reveals **Howell–Jolly bodies.**

Imaging US, abdomen: **spleen** is **absent.**

case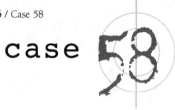

Overwhelming Postsplenectomy Infection

Differential

Sepsis

HIV

Primary Immunodeficiency

Discussion

Patients who have undergone **splenectomy or** who are **functionally asplenic** are at increased **risk for overwhelming bacteremia;** pathogens include **organisms that possess a polysaccharide capsule,** such as meningococcus, *Staphylococcus*, the DF2 bacillus, and especially, *Streptococcus pneumoniae* and *Haemophilus influenzae* type B. Such **functionally asplenic** patients include individuals with **sickle cell disease** and those who have undergone **splenic irradiation. Pneumococcal vaccine** is indicated in all patients who have undergone splenectomy, particularly children and adolescents.

Treatment

Pneumococcal vaccine and prophylactic antibiotics (penicillin, amoxicillin, TMP-SMX).

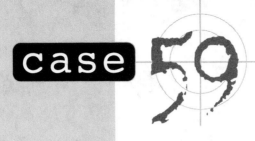

case 59

ID/CC   A 12-year-old girl arrives in the emergency room with **pain, swelling, and limited motion** of her left hand; she also complains of fever and chills.

HPI   The girl was **bitten by a cat** yesterday while playing at a friend's house.

PE   Hand is erythematous, **shiny**, and **markedly edematous**; on palpation, the hand is **tender** with fluctuation (cellulitis); limited passive and active motion; yellowish-green **purulent fluid** drains from the wound; left epitrochlear and axillary **lymphadenitis** without lymphangitis.

Labs   **Gram-negative rods with bipolar staining** of abscess aspirate; **catalase and oxidase positive**.

case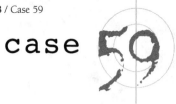

Pasteurella multocida

Differential

Cellulitis

Cat-scratch Disease

Osteomyelitis

Discussion

Pasteurella multocida is the most common bacterium isolated from cat bite wounds and may progress to **osteomyelitis.** Human bite infections are most commonly caused by *Eikenella corrodens* and are treated with penicillin.

Breakout Point

Zoonotic Bacteria: Bugs From Your Pet
Brucella
Francisella
Yersinia
Pasteurella

Treatment

Incision and drainage. Local wound care; **tetanus** and **rabies prophylaxis; polymicrobial antibiotic coverage** with amoxicillin-clavulanate or tetracyclines; meticulous follow-up evaluation for complications.

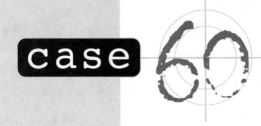
case 60

ID/CC A 28-year-old **sexually active woman** presents with crampy **lower abdominal pain**, yellowish **vaginal discharge**, and general malaise.

HPI She also complains of continuous low-grade fever and reveals that the **pain** is **exacerbated during and immediately after menstruation** (CONGESTIVE DYSMENORRHEA). She uses a copper **intrauterine device** for contraception.

PE VS: low-grade fever. PE: **lower abdominal tenderness**; bimanual pelvic exam demonstrates **purulent vaginal discharge**, bilateral **adnexal tenderness**, and pain on movement of the cervix (MUCOPURULENT CERVICITIS).

Labs CBC: leukocytosis with left shift. Increased ESR; endocervical swab sent for microscopic exam; staining and culture revealed combined infection with *Neisseria gonorrhoeae* (cultured on Thayer–Martin medium) and *Chlamydia trachomatis* (identified on cell culture, immunofluorescence, and antigen capture assay); **laparoscopy** ("gold standard" for diagnosis) confirmed diagnosis.

Imaging USG: free pelvic fluid, dilated tubular structure in adnexa.

Gross Pathology Erythema and swelling of fallopian tubes on laparoscopy; seropurulent exudate noted on surface of tubes from fimbriated end.

Micro Pathology Endocervical swab reveals increased neutrophils and gram-negative diplococci seen both intra- and extracellularly; cervical biopsy reveals inclusions containing *Chlamydia* within columnar cells.

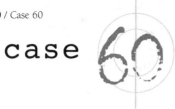

case 60

Pelvic Inflammatory Disease

Differential

Adnexal Tumor
Appendicitis
Endometriosis
Ovarian Torsion
Diverticular Disease
Ectopic Pregnancy

Discussion

Pelvic inflammatory disease usually occurs as a primary infection that ascends from the lower genital tract due to STDs caused by **Neisseria gonorrhoeae** and **Chlamydia trachomatis.** Sequelae of PID include peritonitis; intestinal obstruction due to adhesions; dissemination leading to arthritis, meningitis, and endocarditis; chronic pelvic pain; infertility; ectopic pregnancy; and recurrent PID.

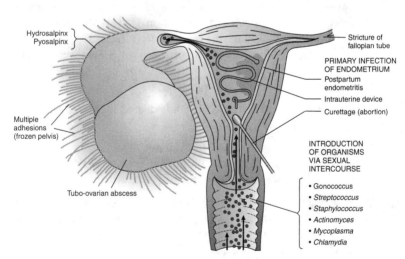

Figure 60-1. Causes and results of pelvic inflammatory disease.

Treatment

Antibiotic therapy with cefoxitin (for *N. gonorrhoeae*) and doxycycline (for chlamydial infection); male partners must be treated for STDs.

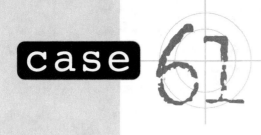

case 61

ID/CC A **20-year-old Asian woman** presents with complaints of **infertility** and **heavy bleeding during menses** (MENORRHAGIA).

HPI She was treated for **pulmonary tuberculosis** a few years ago. She has been unable to conceive despite unprotected intercourse for the past 2 years. Her husband's semen analysis is normal.

PE On pelvic exam, small, fixed **adnexal masses** are palpable that are matted and fixed to the uterus ("FROZEN PELVIS").

Labs Culture of endometrial curettings yields **acid-fast bacilli**; histologic examination of curettings reveals presence of **characteristic tubercles**; Mantoux skin test strongly positive.

Imaging CXR: left apical fibrosis (evidence of old healed pulmonary tuberculosis). (Hysterosalpingography [HSG] is contraindicated in a proven case of tuberculosis. When done in asymptomatic cases, HSG yields certain typical findings, including a **rigid, nonperistaltic, pipelike tube;** beading and variation in filling density; **calcification** of the tube; **cornual block; jagged fluffiness of the tubal outline;** and vascular or lymphatic extravasation of the dye.)

Gross Pathology Tubes are enlarged, thickened, and tortuous; examination of the uterus reveals evidence of **synechiae and adhesions** (leading to **Asherman syndrome**).

Micro Pathology Microscopic exam of tubes, ovaries, and endometrium reveals evidence of **granulomas** with giant cells and **caseation.**

case 61

Pelvic Tuberculosis

Differential

Salpingitis

Tubo-Ovarian Abscess

Endometriosis

Ovarian Mass

Discussion

Genital tuberculosis is almost always secondary to a focus elsewhere in the body, with the bloodstream by far the most common method of spread. The fallopian tubes are the most frequently involved part of the genital tract, followed by the uterus. Ninety percent of patients are cured with chemotherapy, although only 10% regain fertility.

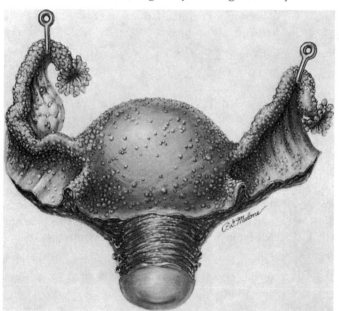

Figure 61-1. Typical specimen of tuberculosis of the reproductive organs as part of generalized tuberculous peritonitis.

Treatment

Four-drug therapy with isoniazid, pyrazinamide, ethambutol, and rifampicin; pyridoxine to prevent isoniazid-induced deficiency.

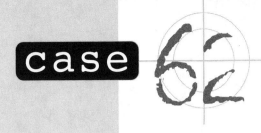

case 62

ID/CC A 25-year-old man complains of **midepigastric pain** that usually begins **1 to 2 hours after eating** and occasionally awakens him at night.

HPI The patient has been diagnosed with **duodenal ulcers** several times in the past, but his **symptoms have** consistently **recurred** even after therapy with histamine (H_2) blockers, antacids, and sucralfate.

PE VS: stable. PE: pallor; epigastric tenderness on deep palpation.

Labs CBC: normocytic, normochromic anemia. Stool positive for occult blood.

Imaging UGI: ulcerations in antrum of stomach and duodenum; antral biopsy specimens yield **positive urease test.**

Gross Pathology Grossly round ulcer (may also be oval) seen as sharply punched-out defect with relatively straight walls and slight overhanging of mucosal margin (heaped-up margin is characteristic of a malignant lesion); smooth and clean ulcer base.

Micro Pathology No evidence of malignancy; **antral biopsies** reveal presence of **chronic mucosal inflammation**; organisms identified on Giemsa stain.

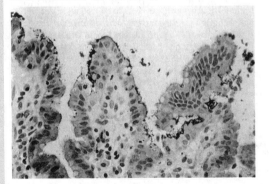

Figure 62-1. High-power view of antral epithelium with severe surface damage resulting from the adherence of large numbers of organisms.

case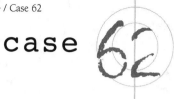

Peptic Ulcer Disease (*Helicobacter pylori*)

Differential

Duodenal Ulcer
Gastric Ulcer
Gastrinoma
Atrophic Gastritis
Gastroesophageal Reflux Disease
Lymphoma

Discussion

Helicobacter pylori grows overlying the antral gastric mucosal cells; 40% of healthy individuals and approximately 50% of patients with peptic disease harbor this organism. Although H. pylori **does not breach the epithelial barrier**, colonization of the antral mucosal layer by this organism is associated with structural alterations of the gastric mucosa and hence with a high prevalence of antral gastritis. Despite the fact that H. pylori does not grow on duodenal mucosa, it is strongly associated with duodenal ulcer, and eradication of the organism in patients with refractory peptic ulcer disease decreases the risk of recurrence.

Breakout Point

Persistent infection with *Helicobacter pylori* is also associated with the development of gastric mucosa-associated lymphoid tumors (MALTomas).

Treatment

Helicobacter pylori eradication employing one proton pump inhibitor (e.g., omeprazole) and two antibiotics (e.g., amoxicillin and clarithromycin).

■ TABLE 62-1 TRIPLE-THERAPY REGIMENS FOR *HELICOBACTER PYLORI* ERADICATION

Regimen	Dose (mg)	Schedule	Days of Treatment	Success Rate	Cost
Proton pump inhibitor	1[a]	b.i.d.	10–14	>90%	$$$$
Clarithromycin	500	b.i.d.	10–14	>90%	$$$$
Metronidazole *or*	500	b.i.d.	10–14	>90%	$$$$
Amoxicillin	2 x 500	b.i.d.	10–14	>90%	$$$$
Bismuth subsalicylate	2 tablets	q.i.d.	10–14	>90%	$ or $$
Tetracycline	500	q.i.d.	10–14	>90%	$ or $$
Metronidazole *or*	250	t.i.d.	10–14	>90%	$ or $$
Clarithromycin	500	b.i.d.	10–14	>90%	$ or $$
Ranitidine bismuth subcitrate	400	t.i.d.	14	>90%	$$$
Clarithromycin	500	b.i.d.	14	>90%	$$$
Tetracycline *or*	500	b.i.d.	14	>90%	$$$
Metronidazole	250	t.i.d.	14	>90%	$$$

[a]Omeprazole 20 mg or lansoprazole 30 mg.
b.i.d., twice a day; q.i.d. four times a day; t.i.d., three times a day.

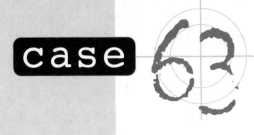

case 63

ID/CC A 9-year-old boy complains of **pain during swallowing** (ODYNOPHAGIA) for 2 days, accompanied by muscle aches, headache, and fever.

HPI He has otherwise been in good health and has no history of cough, runny nose, or itchy eyes.

PE VS: fever. PE: moderate erythema of pharynx; enlarged, **erythematous tonsils** covered with white **exudate**; tender cervical adenopathy.

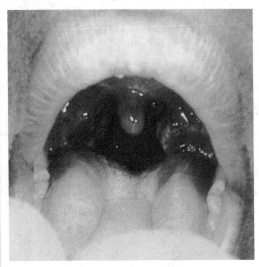

Figure 63-1. Examination of the pharynx in a child shows enlarged, erythematous tonsils with exudate.

Labs CBC: neutrophilic leukocytosis.

Gross Pathology Hyperemia and swelling of upper respiratory tract mucosa; cryptic enlargement of tonsils with purulent exudate; enlargement of regional lymph nodes.

Micro Pathology Acute inflammatory response with polymorphonuclear infiltrate, hyperemia and edema with pus formation; hyperplasia of regional lymph nodes; dilatation of sinusoids.

case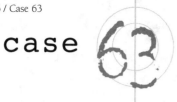

Pharyngitis—Streptococcal

Differential

Infectious Mononucleosis

Viral Pharyngitis

Croup

Foreign Body Aspiration

Ludwig Angina

Epiglottitis

Discussion

Streptococcal pharyngitis is an acute bacterial infection produced by gram-positive **cocci in chains** (*Streptococcus*); pharyngitis is most commonly caused by group A streptococci. Complications due to immune-mediated cross-reactivity and molecular mimicking may include glomerulonephritis and rheumatic fever.

Breakout Point

Features Associated with *Streptococcus* Pharyngitis (Three or Four of the Following Present Makes the Diagnosis More Likely)
• Tonsillar exudates • Tender anterior cervical adenopathy • Fever >100.4°F • Absence of a cough

Treatment

Oral penicillin V.

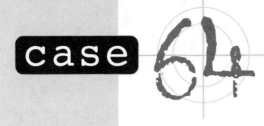

ID/CC A 44-year-old archaeologist presents with **high fever, malaise**, intense **headache, severe myalgia**, and **painful swelling in the inguinal region**.

HPI He recently returned from a trip to **Arizona**.

PE VS: tachycardia; fever. PE: drowsy looking; no meningeal signs; pustule seen at site of an **insect bite** on left upper arm; **inguinal lymph nodes enlarged, fluctuant, and tender** (BUBOES); no lesions on external genitalia.

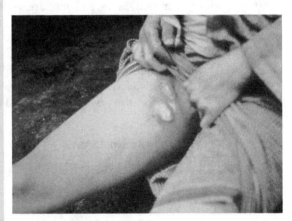

Figure 64-1. Femoral bubo. This plague patient is displaying a swollen, ruptured inguinal lymph node, or bubo.

Labs CBC/PBS: normal; no malarial parasites. Gram-negative bacilli with **"safety pin"** appearance seen in aspirates from buboes.

Gross Pathology Enlarged lymph nodes are necrotic and suppurative; pneumonic form shows lobar consolidation.

Micro Pathology Numerous organisms in suppurative and necrotic lymph tissue.

case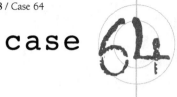

Plague

Differential

Anthrax

Brucellosis

Typhus

Tularemia

Rocky Mountain Spotted Fever

Pasteurella multocida Infection

Discussion

Plague is usually acquired after contact with **rodents and fleas** in endemic areas (southwestern United States). Septic shock, pneumonia, DIC, and vascular collapse are life-threatening sequelae. The **pneumonic form** of the disease has a high fatality rate and requires the institution of **droplet precautions** for hospitalized patients along with prompt administration of **doxycycline prophylaxis** to their contacts.

Breakout Point

Bacterial Shapes

Gull wing—*Campylobacter*
Comma—*Vibrio*
Safety pin—*Yersinia*
Box car—*Bacillus anthracis*
Chinese character—*Corynebacterium diphtheriae*
Tennis racket—*Clostridium tetani*
Lancet—*Streptococcus pneumoniae*
Bean—*Neisseria*

Treatment

Hospitalization with standard precautions; antibiotic therapy with **streptomycin.**

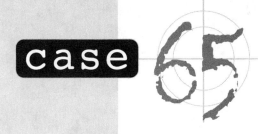

case 65

ID/CC An 11-year-old white boy presents with a high-grade fever, a productive **blood-tinged** cough, **mucoid sputum**, and **pleuritic left-sided chest pain** of a few days' duration.

HPI The child had previously been well and is fully immunized.

PE VS: fever; tachypnea. PE: use of accessory respiratory muscles; central trachea; decreased left respiratory excursion; **increased vocal fremitus in right infrascapular area with dullness to percussion; bronchial breathing** with coarse crackles heard over right lung area.

Labs CBC: increased WBC count; preponderance of neutrophils. ABGs: hypoxemia without hypercapnia. **Gram-positive diplococci in sputum;** α-hemolytic colonies of gram-positive diplococci on blood agar culture.

Imaging CXR: **homogenous opacification of right lower lobe** (LOBAR CONSOLIDATION) with small right pleural effusion.

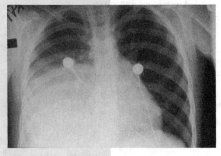

Figure 65-1. Right lower lobe infiltrate with moderate pleural effusion in a child with fever, cough, and localized decreased breath sounds.

Gross Pathology Consolidation of lung parenchyma passes through four stages: congestion and edema, red hepatization, gray hepatization, and resolution.

Micro Pathology Vascular dilatation with hyperemia and alveolar edema; PMNs rich in purulent exudate; fibrin deposition; hardening of lung parenchyma with fibrin clotting inside alveoli (consolidation).

case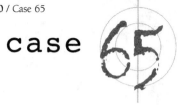

Pneumococcal Pneumonia

Differential

Klebsiella Pneumonia

Legionellosis

Lung Abscess

Influenza

Pulmonary Embolism

Pericarditis

Discussion

Streptococcus pneumoniae is the most common cause of community-acquired pneumonia and produces typical lobar pneumonia. Predisposing conditions include prior splenectomy or nonfunctional spleen, HIV infection, sickle cell anemia, and alcoholism.

Breakout Point

Common Causes of Pneumonia in Various Populations

Neonates—group B streptococci
Adults (age 18–40)—*Mycoplasma pneumoniae*
Elderly (age >65)—*Streptococcus pneumoniae*
Alcoholics—*Klebsiella* (aspiration)
COPD patients—*Haemophilus influenzae*
Cystic fibrosis patients—*Pseudomonas*
HIV-positive—*Pneumocystis carinii*
Taxidermists—*Coxiella, Bacillus anthracis*
Bird handlers—*Chlamydia psittaci*
Immunocompromised—*Aspergillus,* CMV, *Mycobacterium tuberculosis*
Exposure to air conditioners—*Legionella*
Spelunkers (cave divers)—*Histoplasma capsulatum*

Treatment

Parenteral antibiotic therapy; empiric initial choice of ceftriaxone and/or azithromycin followed by culture sensitivity–guided treatment; supportive respiratory therapy; monitoring with clinical and radiologic response.

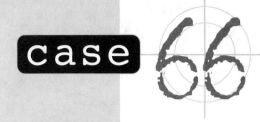

case 66

ID/CC A **10-year-old boy** presents with complaints of acute-onset voiding of **tea-colored urine** and **reduced urinary output.**

HPI The child was treated 1 week ago for **streptococcal pyoderma** that was confirmed by culture. He also complains of puffiness around the eyes and mild swelling of both feet.

PE VS: **hypertension** (BP 140/96 mm Hg); fever; tachycardia. PE: periorbital swelling; mild pitting **pedal edema;** no ascites or kidney mass palpable.

Labs CBC: mild leukocytosis. Elevated BUN and creatinine; **elevated ASO titer;** serum cryoglobulins present. UA: **RBC casts; proteinuria. C3 levels reduced** in blood.

Gross Pathology Smooth, reddish-brown cortical surface with numerous petechial hemorrhages.

Micro Pathology Biopsy shows **diffuse glomerulonephritis** resulting from proliferation of endothelial, mesangial, and epithelial cells; granular, **"lumpy bumpy" pattern** of IgG, IgM, and C3 on immunofluorescence; electron microscopy shows **subepithelial "humplike" deposits** (antigen-antibody complexes).

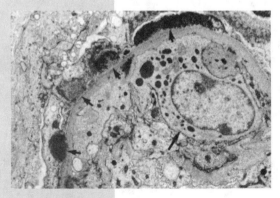

Figure 66-1. Electron micrograph of subepithelial large, irregularly spaced, dome-shaped subepithelial deposits. The deposits are variegated and lie on top of the glomerular basement membrane (*short arrows*). There is endocapillary proliferation with polymorphonuclear neutrophil (*long arrow*) infiltration.

131

case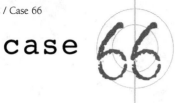

Poststreptococcal Glomerulonephritis

Differential

Goodpasture Syndrome

Lupus Nephritis

IgA Nephropathy

Thin Membrane Disease

Urinary Tract Infection

Discussion

Poststreptococcal glomerulonephritis is a classic immune complex–mediated entity that is associated with acute nephritic syndrome, which develops following infection with nephritogenic group A **β-hemolytic streptococci** (e.g., types 1, 4, and 12, which are associated with pharyngitis, and types 49, 55, and 57, which are associated with impetigo).

Treatment

Penicillin if still infected with *Streptococcus*; diuretics, salt and water restriction, and antihypertensives.

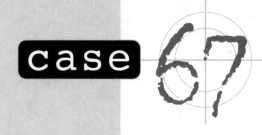

ID/CC A **25-year-old man** presents with complaints of sudden-onset **fever** and chills, urgency and burning on micturition (DYSURIA), and perineal pain.

HPI His symptoms developed a day after he underwent **urethral dilatation** for a stricture.

PE VS: fever. PE: suprapubic tenderness; rectal exam reveals asymmetrically **swollen,** firm, markedly **tender, hot prostate;** prostatic massage is avoided owing to risk of inducing bacteremia; epididymitis and extreme pain.

Labs Examination and culture of urine and prostatic secretions reveal infection with *Escherichia coli.*

Gross Pathology Edematous gland enlargement with suppuration of the entire gland, possibly abscesses and focal areas of necrosis that have coalesced.

Micro Pathology Initially minimal leukocytic infiltration of stroma. Later, necrosis of the gland may lead to gland fibrosis.

case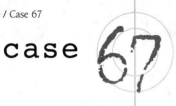

Prostatitis—Acute

Differential	Perianal Abscess
	Urethral Stricture
	Urinary Tract Infection
	Urinary Tract Obstruction
Discussion	*Escherichia coli* **is the most common cause** of acute prostatitis; many cases **follow** the use of **instrumentation for the urethra** and prostate (e.g., catheterization, cystoscopy, urethral dilatation, transurethral resection). Remaining infections are caused by *Klebsiella, Proteus, Pseudomonas,* and *Serratia.* Among the gram-positives, enterococcus and *Staphylococcus aureus* are frequent causative organisms.
Treatment	Antibiotic therapy as directed by urine and blood culture sensitivity tests. Abscesses may require surgical drainage.

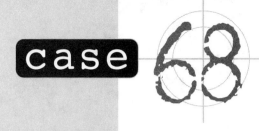

case 68

ID/CC A **65-year-old man** complains of **recurrent burning,** urgency, and **frequency of micturition,** together with vague lower abdominal, lumbar, and perineal pain.

HPI He also complains of a mucoid urethral discharge. He was previously diagnosed via ultrasound with **benign prostatic hypertrophy** but does not report any severe symptoms of prostatism; his medical history reveals **frequent UTIs** due to *Escherichia coli.*

PE VS: stable; no fever. PE: rectal exam reveals **enlarged, nodular prostate;** biopsy obtained to rule out carcinoma.

Labs Examination and culture of expressed prostatic secretions reveal leukocytosis and ***E. coli.***

Imaging IVP/voiding cystourethrogram (to rule out underlying anatomic cause): normal.

Gross Pathology Enlarged prostate with nodularity and calculi.

Micro Pathology Chronic inflammation and few PMNs around glands and ducts on biopsy; dilated ducts containing inspissated secretions (CORPORA AMYLACEA).

case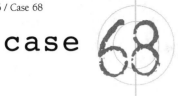

Prostatitis—Chronic

Differential

Benign Prostatic Hyperplasia
Prostate Cancer
Urethral Stricture
Urinary Tract Infection
Urinary Tract Obstruction

Discussion

Bacterial prostatitis is usually caused by the same gram-negative bacilli that cause UTIs in females; 80% or more of such infections are caused by *E. coli*. Chronic bacterial prostatitis is **common in elderly males** with prostatic hyperplasia and is a frequent cause of recurrent UTIs in males (most antibiotics poorly penetrate the prostate; hence the bacteria are not totally eradicated and continuously seed the urinary tract).

▨ TABLE 68-1 LOCALIZATION OF MALE GENITOURINARY INFECTIONS BY SEGMENTAL CULTURE TECHNIQUES

	VB1 (Voided Bladder 1)	VB2 (Voided Bladder 2)	EPS (Expressed Prostatic Secretions)	VB3 (Voided Bladder 3)
How obtained	First 10 mL of voided urine	Midstream sample	Obtained after prostatic massage	First 10 mL of urine after prostatic massage
Significance	Urethral sample	Bladder sample	Prostatic sample	1:100 Dilution of prostatic sample
Urinary tract infection	Abundant leukocytes; positive culture	Abundant leukocytes; positive culture	Abundant leukocytes; positive culture	Abundant leukocytes; positive culture
Urethral infection	Highest colony counts		Lower colony counts	Lower colony counts
Acute bacterial prostatitis	Not generally performed	Leukocytes may be present; culture may be positive; colony counts at $\frac{1}{10}$ level of EPS	Not performed because of danger of septicemia	
Chronic bacterial prostatitis	Little or no evidence of infection	Few to no leukocytes; negative culture	Abundant leukocytes and positive culture	Abundant leukocytes and positive culture
Chronic nonbacterial prostatitis	Negative culture	Negative culture; no leukocytes	Leukocytes present; negative culture	Leukocytes present; negative culture
Prostatodynia			Negative culture; no leukocytes	Negative culture; no leukocytes

Treatment

Antibiotics (TMP-SMX, carbenicillin, quinolones). High fluid intake and abstinence from alcohol. Recurrences are common.

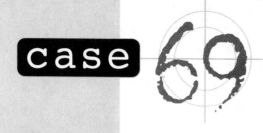
case 69

ID/CC	A 64-year-old man presents with rapidly **progressive dyspnea and fever.**
HPI	He has a history of orthopnea and paroxysmal nocturnal dyspnea and also reports pink, frothy sputum (HEMOPTYSIS). One month ago he underwent a **bioprosthetic valve replacement** for calcific aortic stenosis. He is not hypertensive and has never had overt cardiac failure in the past.
PE	VS: fever; hypotension. PE: bilateral basal inspiratory crackles heard; cardiac auscultation suggestive of **aortic incompetence** (early diastolic murmur heard radiating down the left sternal edge).
Labs	CBC: normochromic, normocytic anemia. Three consecutive blood cultures yield **coagulase-negative** strain found to be **methicillin resistant.**
Imaging	CXR (PA view): suggestive of **pulmonary edema.** Echo: confirms presence of **prosthetic aortic valve dehiscence** leading to incompetence and poor left ventricular function.

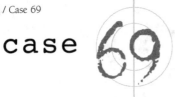

case 69

Prosthetic Valve Endocarditis

Differential Congestive Heart Failure
Aortic Stenosis
Endocarditis
Aortic Regurgitation

Discussion Prosthetic valve endocarditis is subdivided into two categories: early prosthetic valve endocarditis (EPVE), which becomes clinically manifest within 60 days after valve replacement (most commonly caused by **Staphylococcus epidermidis,** followed by gram-negative bacilli and *Candida*), and late prosthetic valve endocarditis (LPVE), which is manifested clinically more than 60 days after valve replacement (most commonly caused by viridans streptococci).

■ **TABLE 69-1 MICROBIAL ORIGIN OF NATIVE AND PROSTHETIC VALVE INFECTIVE ENDOCARDITIS**[a]

Microorganism	Incidence (%)		
	NVE	Early PVE	Late PVE
Streptococci	50	10[b]	30
Viridans	35	—	25
S. bovis	15	—	5
Enterococci	10	—	5
Staphylococci	25	50	40
S. aureus	23	15	10
Coagulase-negative	2	35	30
Gram-negative bacilli	6	15	10
Diphtheroids	—	10	5
Fungi	1	10	5
Other and culture negative	8	5	5

[a]Incidences are approximate; local experience will vary.
[b]Includes all streptococci and enterococci.
NVE, native valve endocarditis; PVE, prosthetic valve endocarditis.

Treatment High-dose parenteral antibiotics—vancomycin (drug of choice for methicillin-resistant *Staphylococcus aureus*), gentamicin, and oral rifampicin; surgical replacement of damaged prosthetic valve; prophylactic antibiotics (amoxicillin) for patients receiving oral/dental treatments to prevent transient bacteremia.

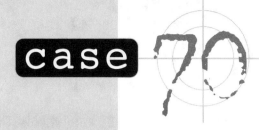

case 70

ID/CC	A 28-year-old black woman who is in her 27th week of pregnancy complains of **right flank pain, high-grade fever,** malaise, headache, and **dysuria.**
HPI	Thus far her pregnancy has been uneventful.
PE	VS: fever. PE: no peripheral edema; **right costovertebral angle tenderness; acutely painful fist percussion on right lumbar area** (POSITIVE GIORDANO SIGN).
Labs	CBC: leukocytosis with neutrophilia. UA: proteinuria; hematuria; abundant WBCs and **WBC casts;** pyocytes on sediment; alkaline pH; **urine culture >100,000 colonies** of *Escherichia coli.*
Imaging	US, renal: CT scan: slightly enlarged kidney.

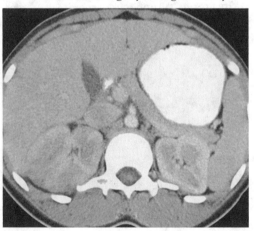

Figure 70-1. Contrast-enhanced computed tomography image shows an enlarged right kidney with several poorly enhancing areas.

Gross Pathology	Kidney enlarged, edematous, and hyperemic with microabscesses in medulla.
Micro Pathology	Pyocytes in tubules; **light blue neutrophils on supravital stain** (GLITTER CELLS); PMN infiltration of interstitium.

139

case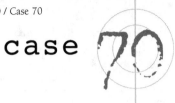

Pyelonephritis—Acute

Differential

Nephrolithiasis

Cystitis

Interstitial Cystitis

Renal Vein Thrombosis

Ureteropelvic Junction Obstruction

Perinephric Abscess

Discussion

An acute bacterial kidney infection caused mainly by gram-negative bacteria such as *E. coli, Klebsiella, Proteus,* and *Enterobacter,* acute pyelonephritis usually results from upward dissemination of lower urinary tract bacteria.

Treatment

Antibiotics according to sensitivity; ampicillin; in nonpregnant patients, fluoroquinolone or ampicillin and an aminoglycoside constitute initial treatment.

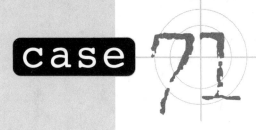

ID/CC A 54-year-old **woman** being treated in the ER is noted to have developed **progressively worsening abdominal pain and high-grade fever with chills.**

HPI She presented to the ER a few hours ago with colicky abdominal pain and was diagnosed with **choledocholithiasis.**

PE VS: **fever** (39.5°C), **hypotension** (BP 80/60 mm Hg); **tachycardia** (HR 120/min). PE: toxic-looking; **icteric**; abdominal exam reveals extremely **tender RUQ with hepatomegaly.**

Labs CBC: **leukocytosis with neutrophilia.** LFTs: **markedly elevated bilirubin, AST, ALT, alkaline phosphatase, and GGT.** Blood cultures grew *Escherichia coli.*

Imaging CT, abdomen: **multiple hepatic abnormalities;** distended gallbladder with perihepatic and pericholecystic fluid collections.

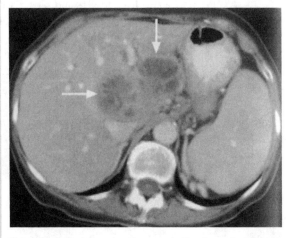

Figure 71-1. Portal venous phase contrast-enhanced computed tomographic scan demonstrates centrally located multiple foci (*arrows*).

141

case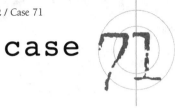

Pyogenic Liver Abscess

Differential

Cholecytstitis

Hepatitis

Hydatid Cyst

Hepatitis

Hepatocellular Carcinoma

Metastatic Tumor

Discussion

A pyogenic liver abscess is a pus-filled cavity within the liver caused by a bacterial infection, typically polymicrobial. The causes of liver abscess include **abdominal infection** such as appendicitis, diverticulitis, or perforated bowel; **sepsis; biliary tract infection;** or **liver trauma** leading to secondary infection. The most common bacteria involved are *E. coli*, *Klebsiella* **spp.**, *Enterococcus, Staphylococcus* **spp.**, *Streptococcus* **spp.**, and *Bacteroides*. Positive blood cultures are found in about half of patients with a pyogenic liver abscess and sepsis is a life-threatening complication. There is significant mortality even in treated patients, and mortality is higher in those with multiple abscesses.

Treatment

Prolonged IV antibiotic therapy; emergent endoscopic (ERCP) or surgical biliary decompression; surgical **drainage** of the **abscesses** if no response to IV antibiotics.

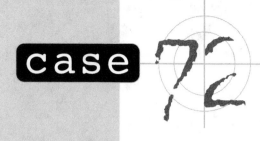

ID/CC A 27-year-old **researcher** presents with sudden-onset **fever,** chills, headache, a **skin rash,** and **painful** swelling of multiple limb **joints.**

HPI Careful history reveals that he was **bitten by a rat** in his laboratory a few days ago; the bite wound has now healed.

PE VS: **fever.** PE: morbilliform **rash** noted over extremities, particularly the hands and feet; **painful swelling** and restriction of movement noted over **both wrist and knee joints.**

Labs CBC: leukocytosis. *Streptobacillus moniliformis* isolated from blood and synovial fluid of inflamed joints; agglutinins to *S. moniliformis* demonstrated in significant titers.

case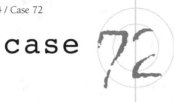

Rat Bite Fever

Differential

Colorado Tick Fever
Relapsing Fever
Typhoid Fever
Collagen Vascular Disease
Miliary Tuberculosis
Collagen Vascular Disease

Discussion

Rat bite fever, which is caused by **S. moniliformis,** is an acute febrile illness that is usually accompanied by a skin rash; **most cases result from the bites of wild or lab rats,** although mice, squirrels, weasels, dogs, and cats may also transmit the disease by bites or scratches. Rat bite fever can also be caused by *Spirillum minus,* with a slightly different presentation. The disease is called **Haverhill fever** when *S. moniliformis* is transmitted by drinking rat excrement–contaminated milk. Distribution is probably worldwide, with most cases occurring in crowded cities characterized by poor sanitation.

■ TABLE 72-1 CLINICAL FEATURES OF RAT BITE FEVER

Streptobacillus moniliformis Streptobacillary Form	*Streptobacillus moniliformis* Haverhill Fever Form	*Spirillum minus*
Incubation period of 1–10 days (usually <7)	Incubation period of 1–3 days	Incubation period 14–18 days
Fever	Fever	Induration at site of inoculation
Chills	Chills	Lesion may progress to ulcer and eschar
Headache	Rash	Fever
Vomiting	Arthritis	Chills
Maculopapular rash (2–4 days after disease onset; rash may become petechial or purpuric and desquamate)	Upper respiratory illness	Regional lymphadenopathy (common)
Septic arthritis	Gastrointestinal complaints	Relapses (common)
Lymphangitis, lymphadenitis (rare)		Rash: purple to red-brown with occasional indurated erythematous plaques
Endocarditis		Severe diarrhea (common)
Pneumonia		Weight loss (common)
Relapses (rare)		Anemia (common)
		Meningitis
		Endocarditis
		Myocarditis
		Nephritis
		Hepatitis

Treatment

Amoxicillin-clavulanic acid (**doxycycline** can also be used).

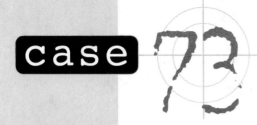

case 73

ID/CC   A 30-year-old man who lives in the **western part of the United States** presents with **high fever**, shaking **chills**, severe headache, myalgias, and diarrhea.

HPI   He reports having had **similar symptoms 10 days ago** that lasted for 4 to 5 days, followed by defervescence accompanied by drenching sweats and marked prostration. He had been **hiking in a tick-infested forest** until about a week before the development of symptoms.

PE   VS: **fever.**

Labs   **Spirochetes found on thick smears of peripheral blood** obtained during febrile periods and **stained with Wright or Giemsa stain.**

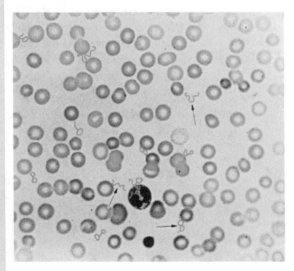

Figure 73-1. Blood smear from a patient shows spirochetes (*arrows*).

case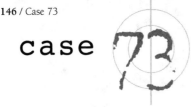

Relapsing Fever

Differential

Leptospirosis

Lyme Disease

Rocky Mountain Spotted Fever

Trench Fever

Colorado Tick Fever

Tuberculosis

Discussion

Relapsing fever is an **acute louse-borne or tick-borne infection** that is caused by blood spirochetes of the genus *Borrelia;* it is characterized by **recurrent febrile episodes separated by asymptomatic intervals.** Unlike other spirochetes, the etiologic agent can readily be detected with Giemsa stain or Wright stain. *Borrelia recurrentis* is the **cause of louse-borne relapsing fever,** whereas a variety of different species produce the **tick-borne disease.** In the United States, the predominant species are *B. hermsii* and *B. turicatae.* Most patients experience the Jarisch–Herxheimer reaction within the first 2 hours of treatment.

Treatment

Doxycycline is the drug of choice (erythromycin may also be used).

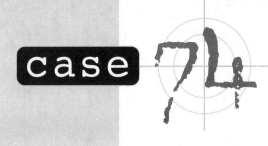

ID/CC A 30-year-old man presents with sudden-onset, crampy **abdominal pain and diarrhea.**

HPI The diarrhea is **watery** and contains **mucus.** The patient also complains of low-grade fever with chills, malaise, nausea, and vomiting. Careful history reveals that he had ingested **partially cooked eggs** at a poultry farm 24 hours before his symptoms began.

PE VS: fever; tachycardia. PE: mild diffuse abdominal tenderness; mild dehydration.

Labs Stool culture yields **pending;** stained stool demonstrates PMNs.

Gross Pathology Intestinal mucosal erythema (limited to the colon) and some superficial ulcers.

Micro Pathology Mixed inflammatory infiltrate in mucosa; superficial epithelial erosions.

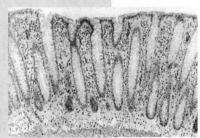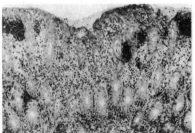

Figure 74-1. The histologic appearance of the mucosa in acute self-limited colitis. In acute self-limited colitis, there is no distortion of crypt architecture.

case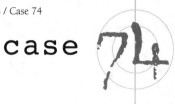

Salmonella Food Poisoning

Differential	Diverticular Disease Botulism Viral Gastroenteritis Shigellosis *Staphylococcus aureus* Food Poisoning
Discussion	*Salmonella* infection is acquired through the ingestion of food (**eggs, meat, poultry**) or water contaminated with animal or human feces; individuals with **low gastric acidity** are also susceptible.
Treatment	Fluid and electrolyte replacement therapy; **antibiotics withheld,** as they **prolong carrier state.** Antibiotic therapy only for malnourished, severely ill, bacteremic, and sickle cell disease patients.

case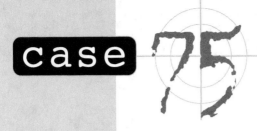

ID/CC	A 14-year-old boy who is known to have **sickle cell anemia** presents with throbbing **pain, redness,** and **swelling** of the **left knee.**
HPI	The patient also complains of fever and chills of 1 week's duration. He has a few **pet turtles** at home.
PE	VS: **fever;** tachycardia. PE: pallor; redness, swelling, and tenderness over left knee; effusion demonstrated in left knee joint; limitation of range of motion of left knee.
Labs	CBC: leukocytosis; elevated ESR. PBS: irreversible **sickling;** blood culture pending organisms also isolated from pus aspirated from left knee (diagnostic of **osteomyelitis**).
Imaging	Nuc: **increased uptake in left tibia.** XR (usually normal during the first 10 days of illness) may reveal changes of bone resorption, detached necrotic cortical bone (SEQUESTRUM), and laminated periosteal new-bone formation (INVOLUCRUM).

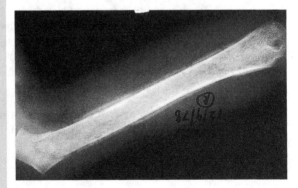

Figure 75-1. Note the periosteal elevation (one of the earlier bony changes).

Gross Pathology	Dense, pale, sclerotic-appearing area in shaft.
Micro Pathology	Changes include suppurative and ischemic destructive necrosis, fibrosis, and ultimate bone repair.

149

case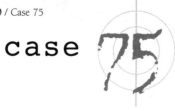

Salmonella Septicemia with Osteomyelitis

Differential

Cellulitis

Sickle Cell Crisis

Arthritis

Deep Vein Thrombosis

Discussion

A striking association has been noted between diseases producing hemolysis (e.g., sickle cell anemia, malaria, and bartonellosis) and *Salmonella* infections; elderly patients with impaired host defense mechanisms, those with hepatosplenic schistosomiasis, and AIDS patients are also at increased risk of severe and recurrent *Salmonella* bacteremia. *Salmonella* osteomyelitis in sickle cell patients presents primarily in young individuals and typically affects long bones. It is believed that the functionally asplenic state found in most sickle cell patients contributes to the increased prevalence of *Salmonella* osteomyelitis.

Breakout Point

> Important note: *Staphylococcus aureus* is still the most common cause of osetomyelitis in patients with sickle cell disease; however, if a patient has *Salmonella* osteomyelitis he or she is more likely to have sickle cell disease.

Treatment

Parenteral antibiotics, with **fluoroquinolones** being first-line agents (**third-generation cephalosporins** may also be used).

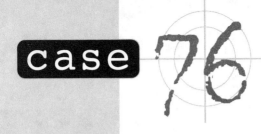

case 76

ID/CC A **2-month-old** girl presents with extensive **bullae** and large areas of denuded skin.

HPI Her mother had suffered from **staphylococcal mastitis** 1 week ago.

PE VS: fever. PE: large areas of red, painful, denuded skin on periorbital and peribuccal areas; flaccid bullae with **easy dislodgment of epidermis under pressure** (NIKOLSKY SIGN); mucosal surfaces largely uninvolved.

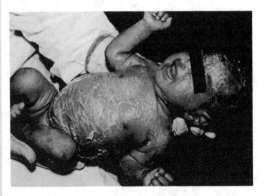

Figure 76-1. Extensive deroded skin on patient.

Labs Vesicle fluid sterile; *Staphylococcus aureus* on blood culture.

case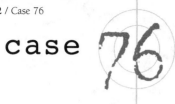

Scalded Skin Syndrome

Differential

Cellulitis

Chemical Burn

Erysipelas

Impetigo

Scarlet Fever

Contact Dermatitis

Discussion

Scalded skin syndrome is caused by the exfoliating effect of **staphylococcal exotoxin.** The action of the exotoxin is to degrade desmoglein in desmosomes in the skin.

Treatment

IV penicillinase-resistant penicillin (e.g., nafcillin, oxacillin). Treat with erythromycin if the patient is allergic to penicillin.

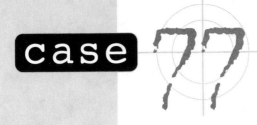

case 77

ID/CC A 10-year-old white girl complains of difficulty swallowing, pain in both ears, and fever of 1 week's duration; she also complains of an extensive skin rash.

HPI The child is fully immunized and has been well until now.

PE VS: fever. PE: **extensive erythematous rash** ("GOOSE-PIMPLE SUNBURN") on neck, groin, and axillae; desquamation and **peeling of fingertips;** circumoral pallor; **lines of hyperpigmentation with tiny petechiae** (PASTIA SIGN) in antecubital fossae; **bright red lingual papillae superimposed on white coat** ("STRAWBERRY TONGUE"); pharyngitis with exudative tonsillitis; cervical lymphadenopathy; normal eardrums.

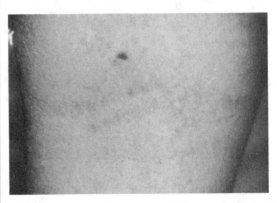

Figure 77-1. PASTIA SIGN in antecubital fossae of the patient.

Labs CBC: leukocytosis with neutrophilia. **Group A β-hemolytic** *Streptococcus pyogenes* on throat swab and culture.

Micro Pathology Toxin-induced vasodilation; inflammatory polymorphonuclear epidermal infiltrate; interstitial nephritis; lymph node hyperplasia.

153

case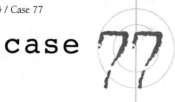

Scarlet Fever

Differential

Mononucleosis
Kawasaki Disease
Measles
Rubella
Scalded Skin Syndrome
Toxic Shock Syndrome
Erythema Multiforme

Discussion

Scarlet fever is a streptococcal infection that is characterized by **morbilliform rash** due to **hypersensitivity to erythrogenic toxin.** Complications include otitis media, pneumonia, glomerulonephritis, osteomyelitis, and rheumatic fever.

Treatment

Penicillin; erythromycin.

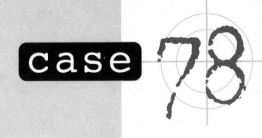

ID/CC　A 36-year-old man executive comes to the emergency room because of the development of **sudden nausea, vomiting, and diarrhea** with **blood and mucus** (dysentery) as well as crampy abdominal pain for 2 days.

HPI　He had just returned from a business trip in **South America**.

PE　VS: low-grade fever. PE: mild dehydration; hyperactive bowel sounds; tender abdomen without definite peritoneal irritation.

Labs　**Leukocytes on stool examination;** organisms isolated on stool culture; on microbiology, organism does not ferment lactose and is **not motile.**

Micro Pathology　Colitis evidenced by severe neutrophilic and mononuclear cell infiltration of lamina propria; ulcers; mucus depletion.

case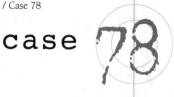

Shigellosis

Differential

Amebiasis

Cholera

Clostridium difficile Colitis

Crohn Disease

Ulcerative Colitis

Yersinia enterocolitica

Discussion

Shigellosis outbreaks occur primarily in areas with **overcrowding** and **poor hygiene** (fecal-oral transmission); **arthritis, conjunctivitis, and urethritis** (REITER SYNDROME) may be complications in HLA-B27–positive individuals. Like *Salmonella, Shigella* causes bloody diarrhea by invading the intestinal mucosa, causing intestinal ulceration and inflammation.

Breakout Point

> The primary virulence factor of *Shigella* (Shiga toxin) is an AB toxin that irreversibly inactivates the 60S ribosome resulting in cell death.

Treatment

Rehydration with antibiotic therapy (TMP-SMX or fluoroquinolone).

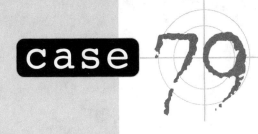
case 79

ID/CC A 56-year-old hospitalized man is found to have an abrupt-onset **high-grade fever** with chills a few hours after he underwent nephrolithotomy.

HPI He was diagnosed with chronic nephrolithiasis with **recurrent UTIs;** a surgery intern also noted **poor urine output.**

PE VS: fever; tachycardia; **hypotension;** tachypnea. PE: confused and disoriented; hyperventilating; diaphoresis; **hands warm** and pink with rapid capillary refill; pulse bounding; on chest auscultation, air entry found to be bilaterally reduced.

Labs CBC: **leukocytosis** with left shift; neutrophils contain **toxic granulations, Döhle bodies,** and cytoplasmic vacuoles; band forms >10%; thrombocytopenia. Prolongation of thrombin time, decreased fibrinogen, and presence of D-dimers (suggesting DIC); raised BUN and creatinine. ABGs: metabolic acidosis (increased anion gap due to lactic acidosis) and hypoxemia (due to **ARDS**). Blood and urine **culture yields gram-negative rods.**

Imaging CXR: evidence of noncardiogenic pulmonary edema (ARDS).

case 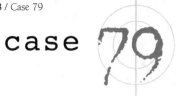 79

Shock—Septic

Differential

Acute Respiratory Distress Syndrome
Anaphylaxis
Disseminated Intravascular Coagulation
Myocardial Infarction
Pulmonary Embolism
Hypovolemic Shock
Acute Renal Failure

Discussion

Almost any bacterium can cause a bacteremia, including *Escherichia coli* (most common), *Klebsiella*, *Proteus*, *Pseudomonas* (associated with antibiotic therapy and burn wounds), *Bacteroides fragilis* (causes of anaerobic septicemias), *Staphylococcus aureus*, *Streptococcus pneumoniae*, and pediatric septicemia due to *E. coli* and *Streptococcus agalactiae*.

Breakout Point

Endotoxin (lipopolysaccharide) is a potent immunostimulant for the development of **septic shock**. This substance, found in the outer membrane of gram-negative organisms, is composed of **lipid A, a core polysaccharide, and O antigen.**

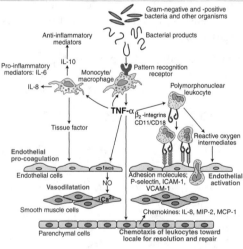

Figure 79-1. Pathogenesis of septic shock. ICAM-1, intracellular adhesion molecule-1; IL-6, interleukin-6; IL-8, interleukin-8; IL-10, interleukin-10; iNOS, inducible macrophage-type nitric oxide synthase; NO, nitric oxide; MCP-1, monocyte chemotactic protein-1; MIP-2, macrophage inflammatory protein-2; TNF-α, tumor necrosis factor-α; VCAM-1, vascular cell adhesion molecule-1.

Treatment

IV antibiotics (with adequate gram-negative coverage); supportive management of multiorgan failure (azotemia, ARDS, and DIC); recombinant human activated protein C for high-risk cases.

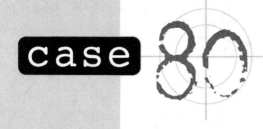

ID/CC A 50-year-old alcoholic white man presents with **fever, abdominal pain,** and rapidly progressive distention of the abdomen.

HPI He was diagnosed with **alcoholic cirrhosis** 1 month ago, when he was admitted to the hospital with jaundice and hematemesis.

PE VS: fever. PE: icterus; on palpation, abdominal tenderness with guarding; fluid thrill and shifting dullness to percussion (due to **ascites**); **splenomegaly**; decreased bowel sounds.

Labs CBC: **leukocytosis.** Ascitic fluid leukocyte count >500/mL; PMNs (350/mL) elevated; ascitic proteins and glucose depressed; gram-negative bacilli in ascitic fluid; *Escherichia coli* isolated in culture; elevated AST and ALT (AST > ALT).

Imaging KUB: ground-glass haziness (due to ascites); no evidence of free air. US, abdomen: cirrhotic shrunken liver; **ascites; splenomegaly; increased portal vein diameter and flow.** EGD: esophageal varices.

Gross Pathology Fibrinopurulent exudate covering surface of peritoneum; fibrosis may lead to formation of adhesions.

Micro Pathology PMNs and fibrin on serosal surfaces in various stages with presence of granulation tissue and fibrosis.

case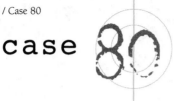

Spontaneous Bacterial Peritonitis

Differential

Abdominal Aneurysm

Appendicitis

Mesenteric Ischemia

Urinary Tract Infection

Pyelonephritis

Perforated Viscus

Discussion

The spontaneous or primary form of peritonitis occurs in patients with advanced chronic liver disease and concomitant ascites; *E. coli* is the most common cause of secondary peritonitis.

Treatment

Treat empirically with a third-generation cephalosporin such as cefotaxime followed by culture sensitivity– guided therapy; long-term prophylaxis with fluoroquinolones may be needed following treatment; supportive treatment for cirrhosis.

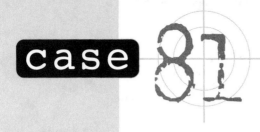

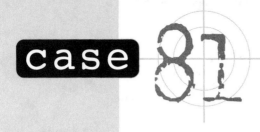

case 81

ID/CC A 25-year-old woman complains of low-grade fever and myalgia of 3 weeks' duration.

HPI She has a history of **rheumatic heart disease** (RHD). One month ago, she underwent a **dental extraction** and did not take the antibiotics that were prescribed for her.

PE VS: fever. PE: pallor; small peripheral hemorrhages with slight nodular character (JANEWAY LESIONS); small, tender nodules on finger and toe pads (OSLER NODES); subungual linear streaks (SPLINTER HEMORRHAGES); petechial hemorrhages on conjunctivae, oral mucosa, and upper extremities; mild splenomegaly; apical diastolic murmur on cardiovascular exam; fundus exam shows oval retinal hemorrhages (ROTH SPOTS).

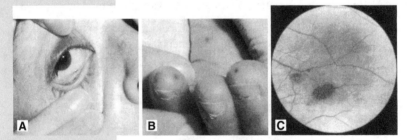

Figure 81-1. A: Conjunctival petechiae. **B:** Petechiae on fingertips; note irregular margins. **C:** Fundus hemorrhage with white center, known as *Roth spot.*

Labs CBC/PBS: normocytic, normochromic anemia. UA: microscopic hematuria. Growth of penicillin-sensitive ***Streptococcus viridans*** on five of six blood cultures.

Imaging Echo: vegetations along atrial surface of **mitral valve.**

Gross Pathology Embolism from vegetative growths on valves may embolize peripherally (left-sided) or to the lung (right-sided).

Micro Pathology Bacteria form nidus of infection in previously scarred or damaged valves.

161

case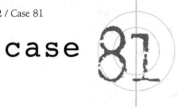

Subacute Bacterial Endocarditis

Differential

Atrial Myxoma

Polymyalgia Rheumatica

Thrombotic Nonbacterial Endocarditis

Liebman-Sachs Endocarditis

Phenaphen Exposure

Vasculitis

Discussion

S. viridans is the most common cause of subacute infective endocarditis, while *Staphylococcus aureus* is the most common cause of acute bacterial endocarditis. Peripheral symptoms such as Osler nodes are believed to result from deposition of immune complexes. Prophylactic antibiotics should be given to all RHD patients before any dental procedure. The disease continues to be associated with a high mortality rate.

Treatment

IV β-lactamase–resistant penicillin and gentamicin; bacteriostatic treatments ineffective.

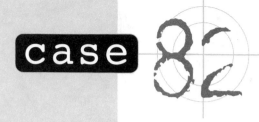

ID/CC A 54-year-old white woman complains of **spiking fever,** chills, **loss of appetite,** several bouts of diarrhea, and **right upper quadrant pain.**

HPI **Ten days ago** she underwent apparently uncomplicated emergency **surgery for suppurative cholecystitis** and was subsequently discharged and sent home.

PE VS: fever. PE: pallor; slight icterus; **pain on percussion of right costal region;** well-healed surgical wound with no evidence of infection; liver not palpable; crepitant rales on right lung base.

Labs CBC: **elevated WBC count (17,000/μL) with predominance of neutrophils.**

Imaging CXR: elevated right hemidiaphragm; slight right pleural effusion. US/CT: **complex fluid collection below diaphragm.**

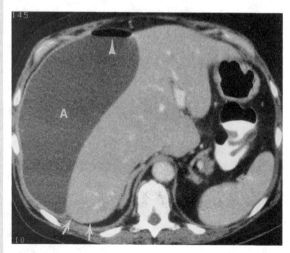

Figure 82-1. A near-water-density collection **(A)** with an air-fluid level (*arrowhead*) in the right perihepatic (subphrenic) space is limited posteriorly by the bare area of the liver (*arrows*).

case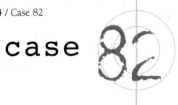

Subdiaphragmatic Abscess

Differential
Pleural Effusion
Pneumonia
Empyema
Tuberculosis
Sarcoidosis

Discussion
Subdiaphragmatic abscess most commonly occurs after abdominal surgery, mainly with septic emergency procedures; it typically presents 1 week or more postoperatively.

Treatment
Percutaneous drainage under ultrasonic or fluoroscopic guidance followed by regular blood and radiologic exams; surgical exploration and drainage.

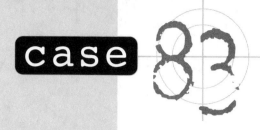

ID/CC A 6-week-old boy, the son of a **prostitute**, is brought to the family doctor because of persistent, sometimes **bloody mucopurulent nasal discharge, anal ulcers,** and a generalized **rash.**

HPI The child was delivered at home, and the mother did not receive any prenatal care.

PE Weak-looking, **icteric** infant with hoarse cry; does not move right limb (**pseudoparalysis**); bloody purulent discharge evident at nares; generalized lymphadenopathy; hepatosplenomegaly; **maculopapular rash** with desquamation on back and buttocks; **bullae on hands and feet.**

Labs CBC: anemia. **VDRL** in both mother and child **positive**; direct hyperbilirubinemia; negative Coombs test;

Imaging XR, plain: periostitis of long bones; bilateral moth-eaten lesions; focal defect in proximal tibial epiphysis with increased density of epiphyseal line (WIMBERGER SIGN).

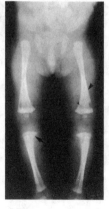

Figure 83-1. Symmetric periostitis (*large arrow*); radiolucent metaphyseal area of osteochondritis (*small arrowhead*); bilateral metaphyseal defects on the upper medial aspect of the tibia; and Wimberger sign (*large arrowhead*). Similar changes may occur at the upper ends of the humeri.

Gross Pathology Pathologic features seen if neonatal disease is left untreated include syphilitic chondritis and rhinitis (causes **saddle-nose deformity**), pathologic fractures, **bowing of the tibia** (SABER SHIN), **V-shaped incisors** (HUTCHINSON TEETH), multicuspid molars (MULBERRY MOLARS), interstitial keratitis, and deafness.

case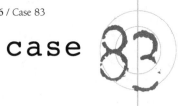

Syphilis—Congenital

Differential

Congenital Toxoplasmosis
Congenital Rubella
Congenital Cytomegalovirus
Congenital Parvovirus
Listeria Infection
Trisomy
Amniotic Bands

Discussion

Treponema pallidum is a spirochete; in-utero vertical transmission occurs from an infected mother to the fetus. Congenital syphilis occurs maximally during 16 to 36 weeks of gestation and may be the cause of stillbirth. It is preventable if the mother has received adequate treatment.

Treatment

Penicillin.

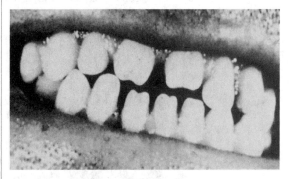

Figure 83-2. Hutchinson teeth in a child.

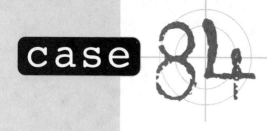

ID/CC An 18-year-old white man presents with a **painless ulcer** on his **penis**.

HPI He admits to having had **unprotected intercourse** with a prostitute 3 weeks ago.

PE **Painless, single, rounded, firm papule with well-defined margins on the dorsal aspect of the glans penis that ulcerates** ("HARD CHANCRE"); nontender, rubbery bilateral inguinal lymphadenopathy.

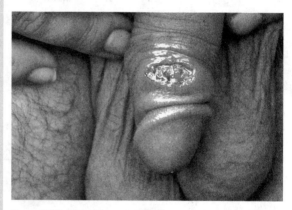

Figure 84-1. Well-demarcated "punched out" painless ulcer on underside of foreskin (chancre).

Labs Treponemes on **dark-field examination** of exudate from chancre; VDRL positive; **FTA-ABS positive**; ELISA for HIV negative.

Micro Pathology Capillary dilatation with plasma cell, PMN, and macrophage infiltration; fibroblastic reaction.

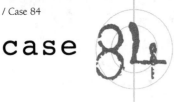

case 84

Syphilis—Primary

Differential

Chancroid
Herpes Simplex
Herpes Zoster
Lymphogranuloma Venereum
Granuloma Inguinale
Superficial Fungal Infection

Discussion

An STD caused by *Treponema pallidum*, a spirochete, primary syphilis is characterized by the appearance of a painless chancre in the area of inoculation. If left untreated, secondary and tertiary syphilis may ensue. Other STDs, such as AIDS, are more prevalent in patients with syphilis

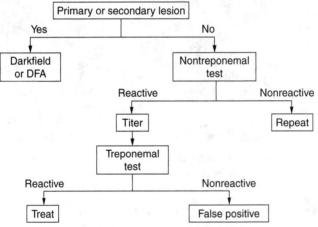

Figure 84-2. Suggested paradigm for the diagnosis of syphilis. Nontreponemal tests are exemplified by the RPR Circle Card Test and the VDRL test, whereas commonly used treponemal tests include the particle agglutination *T. pallidum* (PA-TP) test and the fluorescent treponemal antibody absorbed (FTA-ABS) test. Evaluation of lesion exudates for presence of *T. pallidum* can be performed by darkfield microscopy or direct fluorescent antibody (DFA) staining.

Breakout Point

Painless chancre = syphilis
Painful chancre = *Haemophilus ducreyi*

Treatment

Benzathine penicillin G IM, 2.4 MU single dose.

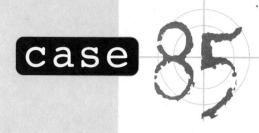

ID/CC A 23-year-old woman presents with a **nonpruritic skin eruption, hair loss,** and generalized fatigue and weakness.

HPI She admits to having had **multiple sexual partners and unprotected sex.** She has had two spontaneous abortions.

PE Extensive **raised, copper-colored, maculopapular, desquamative rash on palms and soles;** generalized nontender **lymphadenopathy** with hepatospleno-megaly; large, pale, **coalescent, flat-topped papules and plaques** in groin (CONDYLOMATA LATA); dull, erythem-atous **mucous patches in mouth;** hair loss (ALOPECIA) in tail of eyebrows.

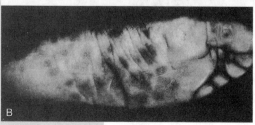

Figure 85-1. A: Vulvar condylomata lata. **B:** Macular rash on sole of foot of same patient.

Labs Skin lesions, mucous patches in mouth, and condy-lomata lata positive for **treponemes; positive VDRL; positive FTA-ABS;** ELISA negative for HIV; CSF VDRL negative.

case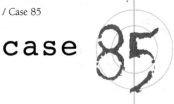

Syphilis—Secondary

Differential	Rocky Mountain Spotted Fever
	Human Papillomavirus
	Disseminated Menigococcemia
	Lymphogranuloma Venereum
	Scabies
Discussion	**Sexual partners must be treated.**

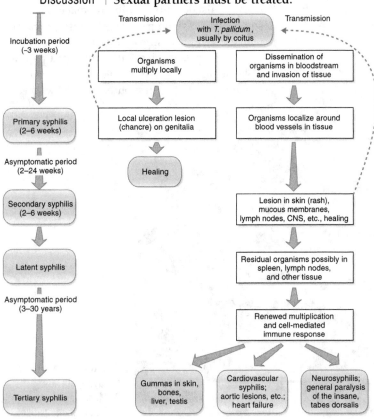

Figure 85-2. Pathogenesis of syphilis.

Breakout Point	Condyloma lata—Secondary syphilis
	Condyloma acuminatum—Human papillomavirus
Treatment	IM benzathine **penicillin G.**

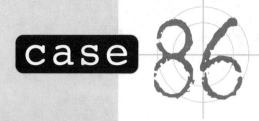

case 86

ID/CC   A 54-year-old man presents with **ataxia, mental status changes,** grossly **deformed ankle joints,** and **shooting pains** in his extremities.

HPI   He remembers having had a "boil" on his penis (PRIMARY SYPHILITIC CHANCRE) many years ago that went away by itself. He also recalls having had a scaling rash on the soles of his feet and the palms of his hands (due to secondary syphilis) some time ago.

PE   Painless **subcutaneous granulomatous nodules** (GUMMAS); **reduced joint position and vibration sense in both lower extremities** (due to bilateral dorsal column destruction); loss of deep tendon reflexes in both lower limbs; loss of pain sensation and **deformed ankle and knee joints with effusion** (CHARCOT NEUROPATHIC ARTHROPATHY); **broad-based gait;** positive Romberg sign (due to sensory ataxia); **pupillary light reflex lost but accommodation reflex retained** (ARGYLL ROBERTSON PUPILS).

Labs   Positive VDRL and **LP: pleocytosis and increased proteins in CSF;** VDRL positive. Normal blood glucose levels.

Imaging   CXR: **"tree-bark calcification" of ascending aorta.**

Gross Pathology   Obliterative endarteritis and meningoencephalitis.

Micro Pathology   Proliferation of microglia; demyelinization and axonal loss in dorsal roots and columns.

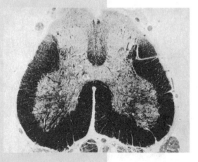

Figure 86-1. Degeneration of the posterior column in the thoracic cord (myelin sheath stain).

171

case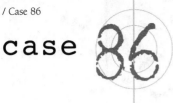

Syphilis—Tertiary

Differential

Lymphoma
Takayasu Arteritis
Tuberculosis
Aortitis
Deep Fungal Infection
Leprosy

Discussion

Tabes dorsalis usually develops 15 to 20 years after initial infection. There may also be visceral involvement (can cause neurogenic bladder).

Treatment

Penicillin.

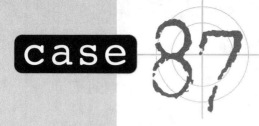

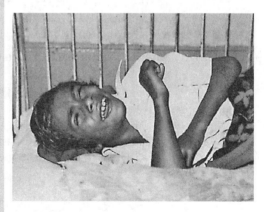

ID/CC	A 12-year-old boy presents with **stiffness of the jaw** and neck along with inability to swallow.
HPI	Twelve days ago he stepped on a **rusty nail,** which produced a small **puncture wound;** the area is now red, hard, and swollen with pus. He has been experiencing tingling sensations and spasms in his calf muscles. He has not received any immunizations within the past 10 years.
PE	**Jaw muscle rigidity** (TRISMUS); **facial muscle spasm** (RISUS SARDONICUS); **dysphagia; neck rigidity;** normal deep tendon reflexes; profuse sweating; patient alert, apprehensive, restless, and hyperactive during PE; loud noise elicits **painful spasms** of the face, neck, abdomen, and back, the latter producing **opisthotonos.**

Figure 87-1. Risus sardonicus with an increased tone of all facial muscles.

Labs	CBC, CSF, blood chemistries normal.
Gross Pathology	There may be fractures of ribs or vertebrae with sustained spasms.

case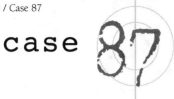

Tetanus

Differential

Tardive Dystonia
Conversion Disorder
Rabies
Mandible Dislocation
Strychnine Poisoning
Dental Infection

Discussion

Tetanus is caused by **tetanospasmin,** a neurotoxin produced by *Clostridium tetani,* an obligate anaerobic, spore-forming, gram-positive rod; the toxin blocks the release of the inhibitory neurotransmitter glycine in the anterior horn cells. Tetanus often occurs in IV drug abusers; neonates of nonimmunized mothers may become infected through the **umbilical cord stump.** The disease may occur even **years** after injury or infection and may also involve the autonomic nervous system (arrhythmias, high/low blood pressure).

Treatment

Surgical débridement of wound; tetanus immune globulin intramuscularly or intrathecally; diazepam; phenobarbital; tetanus toxoid; penicillin IV.

Breakout Point

> The DaPT vaccine is given to children at 2, 4, 6, and 18 months, as well as at 5 years. It protects against diphtheria, tetanus, and pertussis.

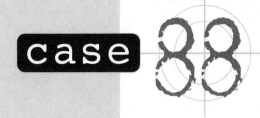

case 88

ID/CC	A 15-day-old **infant** is brought by his mother to the pediatric emergency room in a state of marked **muscle rigidity and spasm.**
HPI	The mother is illiterate and did **not receive any prenatal care**; the delivery was conducted at home, and according to her, was uneventful and full term. The child did **not receive any immunizations**; directed questioning reveals that he has been crying excessively for the past 2 weeks and has not been feeding normally.
PE	Extremely ill-looking infant in a state of **generalized rigidity and opisthotonos**; on slightest touch or noise, spasm worsens and he develops stridor and becomes cyanosed.

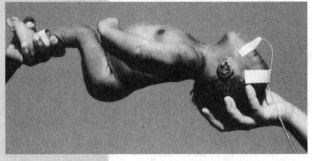

Figure 88-1. Opisthotonos of an infant due to intense contraction of the paravertebral muscles.

Labs	Diagnosis is largely clinical; **culture of umbilical stump yields gram-positive rods with a terminal spore.**

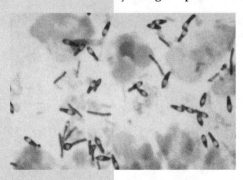

Figure 88-2. Gram-positive rods with oval subterminal and terminal spores.

case 88

Tetanus Neonatorum

Differential

Bacterial Meningitis

Aseptic Meningitis

Dystonic Drug Reaction

Hypocalcemia

Arthrogryposis

Discussion

Tetanus neonatorum accounts for a considerable proportion of infant deaths in developing countries, primarily owing to the **lack of availability of good prenatal care** (no tetanus immunization); untrained birth attendants in rural areas use **contaminated** material to cut or anoint the **umbilical cord**. Tetanus is caused by *Clostridium tetani*, a gram-positive, motile, nonencapsulated, anaerobic, spore-bearing bacillus; its effects are mediated through production of a powerful **neurotoxin (tetanospasmin)**. The toxin acts principally on the spinal cord, altering normal control of the reflex arc by suppressing the inhibition regularly mediated by the internuncial neurons.

Treatment

Ventilatory assistance; supportive management; maintenance of nutritional, fluid, and electrolyte balance; **human tetanus immunoglobulin** for neutralizing unbound toxin; antibiotics such as **penicillin** or **metronidazole** to stop toxin production by killing the organism; control of tetanic spasms with diazepam.

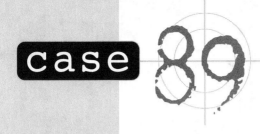

case 89

ID/CC A 30-year-old **woman** presents to the ER with an abrupt-onset **high fever, vomiting, profuse diarrhea,** severe muscle aches, and disorientation.

HPI One day ago she developed an **extensive skin rash** all over her body. Her husband says she used a **vaginal sponge** for contraception.

PE VS: fever; tachycardia; hypotension. PE: extremely toxic-looking; drowsy but responding to verbal commands; **extensive scarlatiniform rash** seen involving entire body; pharyngeal, conjunctival, and vaginal mucosa congested (frank hyperemia); no neck rigidity or Kernig sign demonstrable; funduscopic exam normal; no localizing neurologic deficits.

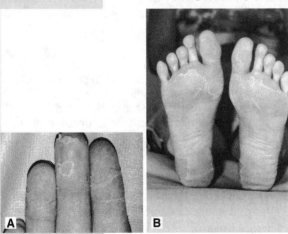

Figure 89-1. A: Desquamation of the palmar surface of the fingers. **B:** Desquamation of the soles.

Labs CBC: leukocytosis; thrombocytopenia. UA: mild pyuria (in absence of UTI). BUN and creatinine elevated; blood cultures sterile; **culture of cervical secretions grows *Staphylococcus aureus*.** LP: CSF normal. Serology for Rocky Mountain spotted fever, leptospirosis, and measles negative.

177

case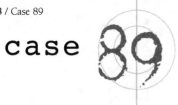

Toxic Shock Syndrome (TSS)

Differential

Scalded Skin Syndrome

Meningococcemia

Necrotizing Fasciitis

Kawasaki Disease

Rocky Mountain Spotted Fever

Discussion

Toxic shock syndrome results from infection with *Staphylococcus aureus*. Its effects are mediated through the **exotoxin TSST-1,** which functions as a superantigen, stimulating the production of interleukin-1 and tumor necrosis factor. Staphylococcal TSS has been associated with the use of **vaginal contraceptive sponges** and with many types of localized staphylococcal soft tissue infections. Most cases of TSS occur in **menstruating women.**

Breakout Point

> **Superantigens** possess potent immunostimulatory properties and the ability to cross-link MHC class II molecules with T-cell receptors. This results in proliferation and cytokine production in T-cells with a massive uncontrolled immune response to the trigger.

Treatment

Vigorous IV fluids and parenteral **penicillinase-resistant penicillin** or first-generation cephalosporins; the patient in this case recovered, and typical skin desquamation was seen over palms and soles during convalescence.

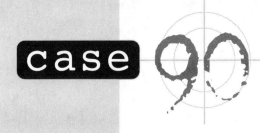

case 90

ID/CC A **6-year-old boy** is brought to the ER in a **delirious state** with fever and marked **dyspnea** that have rapidly progressed over the past 2 days.

HPI His **mother** is an **Asian immigrant**. He has had a low-grade **fever**, cough, **malaise**, and **night sweats** for the past 2 months.

PE VS: fever; tachycardia; marked tachypnea; hypotension. PE: toxic and stuporous; pallor; **central cyanosis**; extensive rales and rhonchi bilaterally; hepatosplenomegaly; lymphadenopathy; funduscopy reveals **choroidal tubercles.**

Labs CBC: **lymphocytosis**; normochromic, normocytic anemia. **Increased ESR; Mantoux skin test positive;** staining and culture of transbronchial and bone marrow biopsy specimens reveal presence of **acid fast bacilli;** ELISA for HIV negative.

Imaging CXR/CT: soft, **uniformly distributed fine nodules throughout both lung fields** (MILIARY MOTTLING).

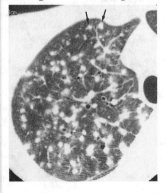

Figure 90-1. Numerous well-defined 1- to 2-mm nodules throughout the lung.

Gross Pathology Myriad 1- to 2-mm **granulomas** demonstrable in lungs, liver, and bone marrow biopsy specimens.

Micro Pathology **Granulomas** with **central caseous necrosis** surrounded by epithelial cells, Langerhans cells, lymphocytes, plasma cells, and fibroblasts in affected tissues.

case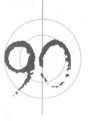

Tuberculosis—Miliary

Differential
Actinomycosis
Septic Arthritis
Brucellosis
Histoplasmosis
Chronic Granulomatous Disease
Nocardiosis
Aspergillosis

Discussion
Miliary tuberculosis results from **widespread hematogenous dissemination** and often presents with a perplexing fever, dyspnea, anemia, and splenomegaly; the disease is **more fulminant in children** than in adults.

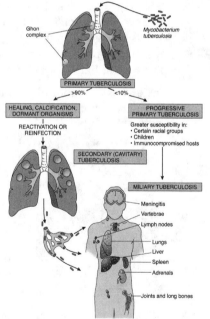

Figure 90-2. Stages of tuberculosis.

Breakout Point

A **granuloma** is the hallmark of a **type IV hypersensitivity reaction** and represents a classic T helper-1 (Th-1) response.

Treatment
Multidrug antitubercular therapy with isoniazid, rifampicin, pyrazinamide, and ethambutol or streptomycin; steroids may be indicated.

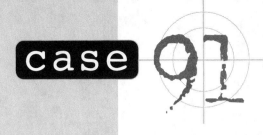

ID/CC A 14-year-old immigrant complains of malaise, **weight loss, fever, and night sweats** of 6 weeks' duration; he also has a mild cough that began to produce **bloody sputum** 3 days prior to his admission.

PE VS: mild fever. PE: **malnourished;** low height and weight for age; bronchial breath sounds with crepitant rales heard over right supramammary area.

Labs CBC/PBS: normocytic, normochromic anemia; WBC count normal with relative **lymphocytosis. Increased ESR;** sputum stained with ZN stain **positive for acid-fast bacilli,** positive MANTOUX TEST.

Imaging CXR: small cavity with streaky infiltrates in right upper lobe; hilar lymphadenopathy; calcified lung lesion (GHON LESION); Ghon lesion and calcified lymph node (RANKE COMPLEX).

Micro Pathology Multinucleated epithelioid **Langerhans cells** surround core of **caseating necrosis** in lung parenchyma, producing fibroblastic reaction at periphery with lymphocytic infiltration and proliferation (TUBERCLE).

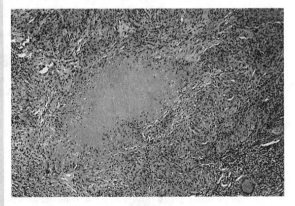

Figure 91-1. Central caseation necrosis with dense macrophage and lymphocyte surround.

case 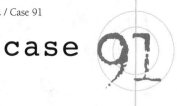 91

Tuberculosis—Pulmonary

Differential

Bronchogenic Carcinoma
Lung Abscess
Lung Metastasis
Histoplasmosis
Lymphoma
Sarcoidosis
Aspergillosis

Discussion

Pulmonary tuberculosis is caused by *Mycobacterium tuberculosis,* an acid-fast, gram-positive aerobic bacillus. An **increasing incidence in AIDS patients** has been observed; drug resistance is becoming common.

Treatment

Multiple drug therapy with isoniazid (INH), rifampin, ethambutol, pyrazinamide, and/or streptomycin.

Breakout Point

Tuberculin skin test (note size = induration only, not erythema).

Cases in which more than 5 mm is regarded as positive:
- People with HIV infection and people receiving immunosuppressive therapy.
- People with recent close contact with a case of pulmonary TB.

Cases in which more than 10 mm is regarded as positive:
- In general, those with chronic illnesses known to predispose to TB and those from areas with a high incidence of TB.
- People with silicosis, malnutrition (including people with gastrectomy or jejunoileal bypass), or diabetes.
- Transplant recipients and people being treated with renal dialysis, corticosteroids, or cancer chemotherapy.
- Children younger than 4 years of age.
- Recent immigrants from high-prevalence areas.
- Medical and laboratory personnel with occupational exposure.
- The poor, especially injection drug users.
- People from prisons, nursing homes, and other group residences.

Cases in which more than 15 mm is regarded as positive:
- People who are generally healthy and not exposed to TB (testing of such persons is discouraged because most positive test results are falsely positive).

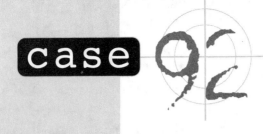

case 92

ID/CC A 12-year-old white boy is brought to his pediatrician because of an **ulcer** on his right thumb together with **swelling of the lymph nodes** in the right axilla with **suppuration**.

HPI He had just returned from summer camp, and upon questioning admits to having played with **rabbits** at the camp's breeding grounds. He has been suffering from **fever**, headache, and muscle aches for almost a week.

PE VS: fever. PE: indurated erythematous nodule with ulcer formation on right thumb; right axillary adenopathy with pus formation; lymphangitis; mild splenomegaly; scattered rales in both lung bases.

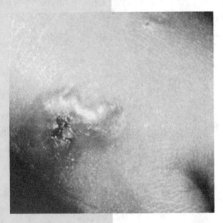

Figure 92-1. Early cutaneous lesion on the thumb.

Labs CBC: **normal WBC count. Increased ESR;** elevated C-reactive protein.

Imaging CXR: bilateral basilar interstitial infiltrates.

Gross Pathology Enlarged, indurated lymph nodes with necrosis and suppuration; skin nodule at site of inoculation with ulcer formation.

Micro Pathology Necrosis and suppuration of lymph nodes; pulmonary and disseminated lesions; **granulomatous nodules** with central caseating necrosis.

183

case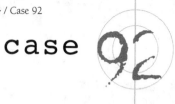

Tularemia

Differential | Psittacosis
Q Fever
Diphtheria
Colorado Tick Fever
Mycotic Infection

Discussion | Tularemia is an acute zoonosis caused by **Francisella tularensis,** a nonmotile, aerobic, gram-negative bacillus; it is transmitted through contact with rabbits, squirrels, or other rodents or tick bites. It may be ulceroglandular, tonsillar, oculoglandular, pneumonitic, or typhoidal.

Treatment | Streptomycin or tetracycline; surgical drainage of fluctuant lymph nodes.

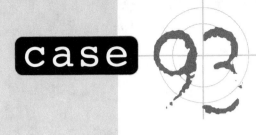

ID/CC	A 27-year-old man is admitted to the hospital for evaluation of **increasing fever** of unknown origin along with malaise, headache, sore throat, cough, and **constipation.**
HPI	He visited Southeast Asia 3 weeks ago but did not receive any prior vaccinations.
PE	VS: **bradycardia**; fever; **fever charting reveals "stepladder" pattern.** PE: mild hepatosplenomegaly; faint **erythematous macules seen over trunk** ("ROSE SPOTS").
Labs	CBC: neutropenia with relative lymphocytosis. **Widal test** positive in significant titers.
Gross Pathology	**Infection of Peyer patches** in terminal ileum leads to necrosis of underlying mucosa, producing longitudinal oval ulcerations.
Micro Pathology	Ulcers bordered by mononuclear cells; typhoid nodules with lymphocytes and macrophages may be present in liver, spleen, and lymph nodes.

case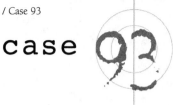

Typhoid Fever

Differential

Abdominal Abscess

Brucellosis

Influenza

Tuberculosis

Tularemia

Lymphoproliferative Disorder

Typhus

Discussion

Because infection is acquired from contaminated food or water, typhoid vaccine is recommended for all those traveling to areas that have had typhoid epidemics. Three vaccines are available: the parenteral vaccine containing the capsular polysaccharide and the oral vaccine containing live attenuated organisms are more effective than the parenteral vaccine containing whole killed organisms. *Salmonella typhi* is transmitted only by humans, whereas all other *Salmonella* species have an animal as well as a human reservoir.

Treatment

Ciprofloxacin or **third-generation cephalosporins;** steroids for severe infection.

case

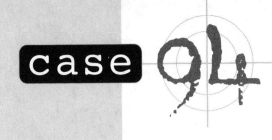

ID/CC A 25-year-old **sexually active woman** complains of **burning on urination**.

HPI She also complains of pain in the lower abdomen and **increased frequency of urination.**

PE Mild suprapubic tenderness.

Labs UA: mild proteinuria; hematuria; WBCs but no casts seen. Urine culture reveals >**100,000** *Escherichia coli* per mL organisms present.

Gross Pathology Infection ascends the urinary tract (urethritis, cystitis, pyelonephritis); mucosal hyperemia and edema.

Micro Pathology Urothelial hyperplasia and metaplasia.

case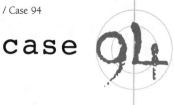

Urinary Tract Infection (UTI)

Differential

Appendicitis

Inflammatory Bowel Disease

Renal Calculi

Urethritis

Endometriosis

Dysmenorrhea

Vulvovaginitis

Pelvic Inflammatory Disease

Discussion

Eighty percent of UTIs are caused by *E. coli*; *Staphylococcus saprophyticus* is the second most common cause. Other causes, in order of frequency, are *Proteus, Klebsiella, Enterobacter, Serratia, Pseudomonas*, and *Enterococcus*; *Chlamydia* and *Neisseria* are also causes of urethritis. Risk factors include female gender, sexual activity, pregnancy, obstruction, bladder dysfunction, vesicoureteral reflux, and catheterization.

Breakout Point

Common UTI Bacteria—SEEK PP	
Serratia	*Klebsiella*
E. coli	*Proteus*
Enterobacter	*Pseudomonas*

Treatment

TMP-SMX; fluoroquinolone for resistant organisms.

■ **TABLE 94-1 QUANTITATIVE CRITERIA FOR IDENTIFICATION OF SIGNIFICANT BACTERIURIA IN SELECTED GROUPS**

Population	Bacteria Counts (CFU/mL)
Asymptomatic bacteriuria	
In women	$\geq 10^5$, usually in two consecutive specimens
In men	$\geq 10^5$
Acute uncomplicated pyelonephritis	$\geq 10^5$
Acute dysuria in women	$\geq 10^2$, with pyuria
Specimens collected by catheter	$\geq 10^2$

CFU, colony-forming unit.

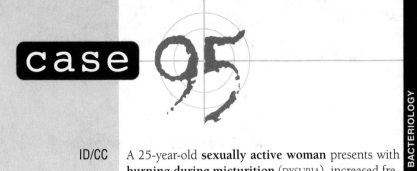

ID/CC   A 25-year-old **sexually active woman** presents with **burning during micturition** (DYSURIA), increased frequency and urgency of micturition, and low-grade fever.

HPI   She is otherwise in perfect health.

PE   VS: fever.

Labs   UA: abundant WBCs; mild proteinuria but no casts; staining of sediment reveals presence of gram-positive cocci. Urine culture isolates **coagulase-negative** *Staphylococcus.*

case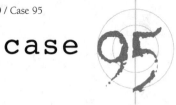

UTI with *Staphylococcus saprophyticus*

Differential Appendicitis
Inflammatory Bowel Disease
Renal Calculi
Urethritis
Endometriosis
Dysmenorrhea
Vulvovaginitis
Pelvic Inflammatory Disease

Discussion Enterobacteriaceae such as *Escherichia coli*, *Klebsiella* species, and *Proteus* and *Pseudomonas* species are the most common organisms causing UTI. After *E. coli*, *Staphylococcus saprophyticus* is the most common cause of primary nonobstructive UTI in sexually active young women.

■ **TABLE 95-1 APPROACH TO TREATMENT OF URINARY TRACT INFECTIONS FOR DIFFERENT CLINICAL PRESENTATIONS**

Type of Infection	Treatment	Rationale
Cystitis	Short course (3 days) preferred	Effective for bacterial cystitis; not effective in patients with early pyelonephritis or resistant bacteria, which are detected by follow-up culture or by relapse of symptoms
Pyelonephritis	10–14 days, full doses; antimicrobial prescription based on susceptibility tests; drug with urinary excretion preferred	Requires antimicrobials that achieve high concentrations in renal tissue as well as urine
Asymptomatic bacteriuria	Indicated only for pregnant women or patients about to undergo traumatic urologic procedures	24%–40% of pregnant women with asymptomatic bacteremia and sepsis likely following procedures with potential mucosal trauma and bleeding
Recurrent or multiple reinfections	Prophylaxis; long term (6–12 months) low dose or postintercourse	Eradicates colonizing flora; repeatedly sterilizes urine
Relapse	Long-term treatment (e.g., 4–8 weeks or longer)	Suggests tissue invasion or structural abnormality and merits investigation

Treatment Antibiotics (ampicillin, cotrimoxazole, or ciprofloxacin).

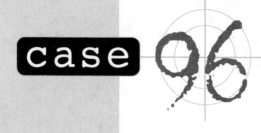

case 96

ID/CC   A 30-year-old man presents with sudden-onset fever, colicky **abdominal pain,** and **watery diarrhea.**

HPI   He had eaten **raw oysters** at a friend's party the day before (incubation period 4 hours to 4 days).

PE   VS: fever; tachycardia. PE: no dehydration; diffuse abdominal tenderness; increased bowel sounds.

Labs   *Vibrio* isolated from stool in a high-salt-content (halophilic vibrio) culture medium; PMNs in stool; **Kanagawa phenomenon** (beta-hemolysis on medium containing human blood; done as an indicator for pathogenicity) **positive.**

case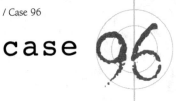

Vibrio parahaemolyticus Food Poisoning

Differential	Botulism
	Viral Gastroenteritis
	Organophosphate Poisoning
	Tetrodotoxin
Discussion	**Seafood** is the main source of the organism. After ingestion, *Vibrio parahaemolyticus* multiplies in the gut and produces a **diarrheal enterotoxin** (Table 96-1 on page nos. 193 and 194).
Treatment	Fluid and electrolyte balance; antibiotics not required (since they do not shorten course of infection).

■ TABLE 96-1 CLINICAL FEATURES OF AGENT-SPECIFIC FOOD-BORNE DISEASE WITH SYMPTOM ONSET OF GREATER THAN 12 HOURS

Organism or Agent	Incubation	Duration of Illness (range)	Diarrhea	Fever	Vomiting	Enterotoxin	Invasion	Foods Most Commonly Implicated	Comments
Salmonella	8–48 h	3 days (1–14 days)	+++	++	+	+	+ (little mucosal damage)	Eggs, poultry, beef, dairy products	Infection with some serotypes can lead to severe complications in certain patients (those with malignancy, atherosclerosis, and AIDS); treatment not recommended except in severe or disseminated disease because it prolongs carriage of organism; stool contains white blood cells and may contain blood
Shigella	24–72 h (up to 7 days)	3 days (1–14 days)	+++	+++	±	+	++	Salads (eggs, tuna, poultry), milk	Low infective dose (10–10² organisms); person-to-person transmission common; stools often contain blood, mucus, and pus; systemic symptoms (headache, malaise, lethargy) common
Yersinia	24–72 h (up to 6 days)	7 days (2–30 days)	+++	++	±	+	+	Milk (raw or chocolate), tofu	Abdominal pain is a prominent feature of illness and may be confused with appendicitis; presence of pharyngitis common in children; rheumatologic postinfectious complications have been reported
Campylobacter	2–11 days	3 days (2–30 days)	+++	++	±	+	+	Raw, milk, poultry, beef, clams, pet animals	Stool contains red and white blood cells; most resistant to trimethoprim-sulfamethoxazole; complications include meningitis and Guillain-Barré syndrome

(Continued)

193

■ TABLE 96-1 CONTINUED

Organism or Agent	Incubation	Duration of Illness (range)	Diarrhea	Fever	Vomiting	Enterotoxin	Invasion	Foods Most Commonly Implicated	Comments
Escherichia coli (entero-toxigenic)	24–72 h	3 days (1–14 days)	+++	+	−	+	−	Salads, peeled fruits, meat dishes, pastries	At least two toxins elaborated: heat labile (similar to choleratoxin) and heat stable; most common bacterial agent of travelers' diarrhea
Vibrio para-haemolyti-cus	4–96 h	3 days (2–10 days)	++	±	+	+	− (not documented in humans)	Oysters, crabs, shellfish, sea water, contam-inated food	Antimicrobials do not shorten illness; fecal white blood cells and blood uncommon
Clostridium botulinum	12–36 h (may be as long as 8 days)	Weeks to months	±	−	±	++ (neuro-toxin)	−	Raw honey (infants), improperly canned food	Neurologic symptoms are results of parasympathetic and neuromuscular blockade; fatality rate 15%; treatment is early administration of antitoxin; infants under 1 year of age should not be fed raw honey
Rotavirus	48–72 h	5 days (3–14 days)	+++	+ (low grade)	++	−	(superficial damage to mucosa)	Fresh water, seafood	Primarily an illness of infants and children; endemic in nature; respira-tory symptoms common; can cause severe dehydration in children
Calicivirus (Norwalk and Norwalklike viruses)	24–48 h	1 day (1–3 days)	++	+ (low grade)	++	−	− (superficial damage to mucosa)	Shellfish, drinking water	Affects primarily older children and adults; endemic in nature

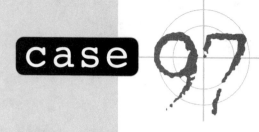

ID/CC   A 35-year-old man presents to the emergency room with high-grade fever, marked weakness, and a hemorrhagic **vesiculobullous skin eruption.**

HPI   He had just returned from deep-sea fishing in the Gulf of Mexico, where he had consumed large quantities of **seafood.** He has been diagnosed with **chronic liver disease** (due to hemochromatosis).

PE   VS: fever; hypotension; tachycardia. PE: icterus; vesiculobullous skin lesions seen on an otherwise-bronzed complexion.

Labs   Blood culture on **high-salt medium** (halophilic bacteria) reveals growth of *Vibrio;* evidence of hemochromatosis (hyperglycemia, hyperbilirubinemia, increased serum iron).

case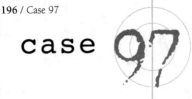

Vibrio vulnificus **Food Poisoning**

Differential

Cholera

Clostridial Gas Gangrene

Hepatitis

Disseminated Intravascular Coagulation

Sepsis

Discussion

Halophilic *Vibrio vulnificus* should be suspected and treated in any individual with chronic liver disease who presents with septicemia and skin lesions 1 to 3 days following seafood ingestion.

Treatment

Ceftazidime and **doxycycline, ciprofloxacin;** supportive.

case 98

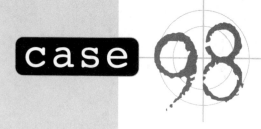

ID/CC A 2-year-old boy is brought to the emergency room because of **paroxysms** and multiple **coughs** in a single expiration, followed by a high-pitched **inspiratory whistle or whoop.**

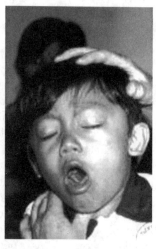

Figure 98-1. Severe paroxysmal coughing.

HPI For the past 2 weeks he has had a runny nose, low-grade fever, muscle pains, and headache. His **immunization schedule is incomplete.**

PE VS: fever. PE: child apprehensive and becomes cyanotic during cough paroxysm; thick green mucus expelled with cough; conjunctival injection.

Labs CBC: **marked leukocytosis with lymphocytosis.** Diagnosis confirmed by culture on Bordet–Gengou medium.

Gross Pathology Small conjunctival and brain hemorrhages may appear during paroxysms; bronchiectasis may also be a complication.

Micro Pathology Signs of acute inflammation in upper respiratory tract mucosa, with erythema, petechiae, polymorphonuclear infiltrate, and necrosis.

case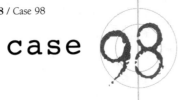

Whooping Cough

Differential | Bronchiolitis
Croup
Respiratory Syncytial Virus Infection
Pneumonia
Epiglottitis

Discussion | A bacterial infection of the upper respiratory tract caused by **Bordetella pertussis,** a gram-negative coccobacillus, whooping cough is transmitted by droplets and comprises three stages: prodromal (catarrhal), paroxysmal (coughing), and convalescent. It is largely preventable with universally administered diphtheria toxoid, tetanus toxoid, and pertussis acellular (DTP) vaccine. Pertussis toxin is a heat-labile exotoxin in which ADP ribosylates the inhibitory G protein, thus inactivating it and leading to constant activation of adenylate cyclase and increased cAMP. The remarkable lymphocytosis is due to pertussis toxin inhibiting chemokine receptors. As a result, lymphocytes are unable to leave the bloodstream.

Breakout Point

> The whooping cough is produced by paroxysmal hacking coughs that end with an inspiratory "whoop" as air rushes over a swollen glottis.

Treatment | Largely supportive; **erythromycin** for treatment of patient and close contacts.

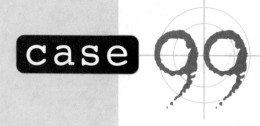

case 99

ID/CC A **14-year-old child** who lives in **tropical Africa** presents with **multiple papillomatous skin lesions and pain in both legs**.

HPI The **first lesion** had appeared on the leg as a **small indurated papule that ulcerated** into a granulomatous papilloma.

PE **Multiple papillomatous skin lesions** seen, especially in intertriginous areas; lesions were painless and exuding a serous fluid; **painful hyperkeratotic lesions** seen on palms and soles; both **tibia were tender** to palpation.

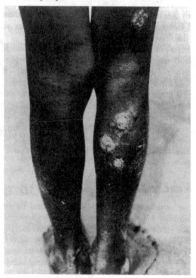

Figure 99-1.
Shallow ulcers on the leg, typical in this condition.

Labs **Dark-field microscopic examination** of exudate from lesions established the diagnosis by revealing organisms with the **characteristic morphology and rotational motion of pathogenic treponemes;** nontreponemal serologic tests (i.e., VDRL and RPR tests) and treponemal tests (i.e., FTA-ABS test) were positive.

Imaging XR, legs: evidence of **periostitis of the tibia.**

199

case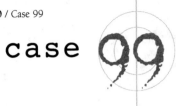

Yaws

Differential

Impetigo
Leishmaniasis
Leprosy
Scabies
Osteomyelitis
Sarcoidosis

Discussion

Yaws, the most common of the nonvenereal treponematoses, is a chronic infection of skin and bones caused by *Treponema pertenue*. Yaws occurs in tropical areas of Africa, Asia, and Central and South America; it is principally a disease of childhood, and initial infection occurs between 5 and 15 years of age. Transmission is by direct contact with infected skin lesions containing treponemes and is fostered by conditions of overcrowding and poor hygiene. The disease may occur in three stages: primary, secondary, and tertiary. Only lesions of primary and secondary yaws are infectious.

Treatment

Long-acting intramuscular **benzathine penicillin G** is the treatment of choice.

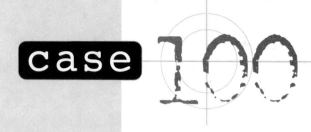

ID/CC A 28-year-old woman complains of **painful swelling of the right knee** and **tender skin eruptions** on both shins.

HPI For the past 2 weeks she has also had **watery diarrhea** that developed after she consumed some **raw pork**. She also complains of low-grade fever and mild abdominal pain.

PE VS: low-grade fever; tachycardia. PE: mild dehydration; swollen and warm knee joint with painful restriction of all movements (ARTHRITIS); multiple **tender, erythematous plaques and nodules** (ERYTHEMA NODOSUM) seen over both shins.

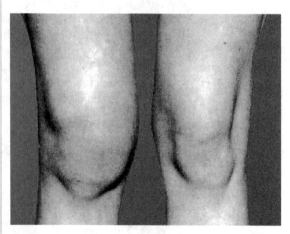

Figure 100-1. Unilateral painful knee effusion is a common clinical presentation in these patients.

Labs CBC: leukocytosis patient is **HLA-B27–positive.**

Micro Pathology Oval ulcers with long axis in the direction of bowel flow, similar to ulcers caused by typhoid fever (intestinal tubercular ulcers are transverse).

case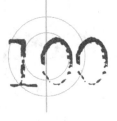

Yersinia Enterocolitis

Differential
Amebiasis
Campylobacter Infection
Clostridium difficile Colitis
Salmonellosis
Ulcerative Colitis
Diverticulitis
Vibrio Infection

Discussion
Yersinia enterocolitica is an invasive gram-negative **intracellular pathogen** that causes **gastroenteritis,** most frequently involving the distal ileum and colon (enterotoxin-mediated), **mesenteric adenitis** (due to necrotizing and suppurative gut lesions) and ileitis **(pseudoappendicitis),** and sepsis; infection may trigger a variety of **autoimmune phenomena,** including erythema nodosum, reactive arthritis, and possibly Graves disease, especially in HLA-B27–positive individuals. Spread is by the fecal-oral route and occurs via contaminated milk products or water, swine, or household pet feces.

Treatment
Supportive; antibiotics (aminoglycosides, fluoroquinolones) indicated in severe infections.

questions

1. A 4-year-old boy develops a painful lump on the left side of his face. Initially, it appears that it is tender to touch. He is brought to the emergency room when his mother notices that there is pus draining from the wound, which now appears to communicate with his oral cavity. A culture is sent from the wound that returns as an acid-fast organism that grows in a filamentous pattern with the presence of "sulfur granules." The most likely organism in this case is:

   A. *Mycobacterium scrofulaceum*
   B. *Nocardia asteroides*
   C. *Bacteroides, Fusobacterium,* and *Treponema* polymicrobial infection
   D. *Mycobacterium marinum*
   E. *Actinomyces israelii*

2. A 23-year-old intravenous drug abuser is brought from the homeless shelter because of a productive cough, chills, and hemoptysis. On physical exam, his temperature is found to be 39.2°C. He has an appreciable 3/6 systolic ejection murmur. He is admitted and blood cultures are drawn. In the interval, he is found to have vegetations on the tricuspid valve by a transesophageal echocardiogram. Which of the following is likely to be found on the patient's blood cultures when they return positive?

   A. *Staphylococcus aureus*
   B. *Staphylococcus epidermidis*
   C. *Streptococcus viridans*
   D. *Staphylococcus saprophyticus*
   E. *Streptococcus pneumoniae*

3. A 23-year-old female complains of a fishy-smelling vaginal discharge. She notes no recent antibiotic use. Furthermore, she notes no vaginal pruritus. Upon presentation to the gynecologist a pelvic exam is performed, and no cervical motion tenderness is noted. A wet mount is prepared of the vaginal discharge, and on visualization, large epithelial cells covered with innumerable bacteria are seen. The patient is placed on antibiotics appropriate for which of the following organisms?

A. *Trichomonas vaginalis*
B. *Chlamydia trachomatis*
C. *Actinomyces israelii*
D. *Candida albicans*
E. *Gardnerella vaginalis*

4. A 4-year-old boy develops a cough and sore throat. His mother decides to soothe the infant's throat by providing him with spoonfuls of unprocessed raw honey. Within a few days, she notes he has become progressively weak and lethargic appearing and he is brought to the emergency room for treatment. Given the history, the ER physician presumes the symptoms are due to which of the following toxins?

A. Tetanus toxin
B. Botulinum toxin
C. Diphtheria toxin
D. Pertussis toxin
E. Cord factor

5. A 30-year-old woman presents to the emergency room with sharp upper quadrant pain. The only relevant past medical history is that she has had numerous sexually transmitted diseases. A work-up ensues, including a chest x-ray, which is stated to be normal, and an ultrasound, which fails to demonstrate the presence of gallbladder disease. She is referred to a gynecologist who performs a laparoscopy that demonstrates the presence of adhesions between her liver capsule and the peritoneum. This can occur as a consequence of infection with which of the following?

A. *Neisseria gonorrhoeae*
B. *Ehrlichia chaffeensis*
C. *Mycobacterium tuberculosis*
D. *Calymmatobacterium granulomatis*
E. *Streptobacillus moniliformis*

6. A 25-year-old man presents to the emergency room with a painful swollen finger. He notes that he cut his finger while out fishing on a commercial fishing boat. He is found to have significant axillary lymphadenopathy. The physician starts the patient on penicillin for a presumed diagnosis of "seal finger." A culture taken of the wound is likely to grow which of the following?

A. *Bartonella henselae*
B. *Francisella tularensis*
C. Orf
D. *Erysipelothrix rhusiopathiae*
E. *Bacillus anthracis*

7. While on a medical mission to Angola, a fourth-year medical student is assigned to work in the makeshift hospital of a refugee camp. He sees numerous cases of severely dehydrated children. He learns that the children have had copious "rice water" stools and cannot tolerate oral hydration, as it causes further diarrhea. He is asked to start intravenous fluids in these children. Stool cultures return positive for *Vibrio cholerae,* which causes life-threatening diarrhea through the elaboration of a toxin with which of the following actions?

   A. Blocks the release of glycine
   B. Blocks the release of acetylcholine
   C. Degrades tissues
   D. Stimulates adenylate cyclase
   E. Inactivates protein synthesis

8. A 16-year-old boy is brought to the emergency room by his parents, as he has been experiencing bloody diarrhea for 1 week. He also complains of not urinating often and the development of a generalized rash. His laboratory studies demonstrate an increased BUN and creatinine as well as the presence of microangiopathic hemolytic anemia. Out of concern for the development of the hemolytic uremic syndrome, he is directly admitted to the intensive care unit for aggressive hydration and intravenous antibiotics. This condition is associated with infection by which of the following?

   A. Enteropathogenic *Escherichia coli*
   B. *Bacteroides fragilis*
   C. Enterotoxigenic *Escherichia coli*
   D. Enterohemorrhagic *Escherichia coli*
   E. Enteroinvasive *Escherichia coli*

9. A 26-year-old pregnant woman begins to experience contractions at 38 weeks' gestation. She is brought to the hospital for delivery. She experiences a complicated prolonged delivery, but ultimately delivers. Her newborn is transferred to the neonatal intensive care unit and is found to have meningitis. Review of the records suggests that the mother was colonized with *Streptococcus agalactiae.* Culture of the infant's cerebrospinal fluid is consistent with *S. agalactiae* meningitis. Which of the following describes the staining characteristic of the organism?

   A. Gram-positive cocci in clusters
   B. Gram-positive rods
   C. Gram-negative cocci
   D. Gram-positive cocci in chains
   E. Gram-negative rods

10. A 14-year-old boy returns from a weekend of camping with his boy scout troop. He spent the August weekend hiking through the woods of Connecticut in shorts. When he returned home, he noted the development of a "bull's eye rash" on his lower leg. Serologic studies demonstrate that he has Lyme disease. Which of the following correctly lists the causative organism as well as the vector that transmits the disease?

    A. *Bartonella bacilliformis* and the sandfly
    B. *Borrelia burgdorferi* and the *Ixodes* tick
    C. *Ehrlichia chaffeensis* and the *Ixodes* tick
    D. *Borrelia recurrentis* and lice
    E. *Borrelia burgdorferi* and the *Dermacentor* tick

11. A 12-year-old boy is brought to the emergency room after being bitten by the family cat. While playing with the cat, the boy sustained a bite and initially hid the wound from his mother. Now, a day later, the boy's hand is swollen significantly. An x-ray of the hand demonstrates puncture of the periosteum of the lower ulna. A hand surgeon is immediately called in for débridement of the wound. Surgical cultures are likely to grow which organisms?

    A. *Spirillum minus*
    B. *Nocardia asteroides*
    C. *Listeria monocytogenes*
    D. *Streptococcus mutans*
    E. *Pasteurella multocida*

12. A 16-year-old boy complains of an exquisitely tender ear. He is the star member of the school's diving team and is concerned that the pain in his ear will affect his performance at the state championships. He is brought to the family physician by his mother, who notes that although his tympanic membrane moves normally with pneumatic otoscopy, it is erythematous. There is a slight amount of purulent discharge in the canal and the exam is poorly tolerated secondary to pain on retraction of the tragus. Suspecting otitis externa, the physician prescribes antibiotic ointment to cover which of the most likely organisms?

    A. *Haemophilus influenzae*
    B. *Mycoplasma pneumoniae*
    C. *Moraxella catarrhalis*
    D. *Staphylococcus saprophyticus*
    E. *Pseudomonas aeruginosa*

13. A 54-year-old man presents to the gastroenterologist with the complaint of heartburn for several years. He notes that his symptoms have been poorly controlled with histamine blockers and antacids. On physical examination, the patient has no significant abnormalities, except for having occult blood detected by guaiac test on his rectal exam. He is scheduled for an endoscopic biopsy of his stomach to evaluate for peptic ulcer disease. However, in the meantime, which of the following tests may be found positive in this patient?

A. Weil–Felix reaction
B. Urease breath test
C. Whiff test
D. Mantoux test
E. Nagler reaction

14. A 68-year-old otherwise healthy male presents to his internist with a fever, blood-tinged sputum, and left pleuritic chest pain for 2 days. On exam, the patient has audible crackles over the left side of his chest as well as dullness to percussion. He notes that his wife was recently sick with a similar illness, and needed antibiotics. A sputum culture is obtained in the office. The most likely organism to cause his pneumonia would appear as:

A. gram-negative kidney-shaped diplococci
B. gram-positive rods with a terminal spore
C. gram-positive lancet-shaped diplococci
D. gram-negative comma-shaped organism
E. gram-negative rods with a mucoid capsule

15. A 3-year-old boy presents to the pediatrician with a honey-crusted rash around his mouth. His mother says that the child has had a low-grade fever. On exam, the child appears well. A culture is taken of the lesion and titers for antistreptolysin O (ASO) are sent. The culture returns with gram-positive cocci in chains and his ASO titers are negative. The patient is placed on antibiotics. His lesions are most consistent with which of the following skin conditions?

A. Scalded skin syndrome
B. Erysipelas
C. Toxic shock syndrome
D. Impetigo
E. Scarlet fever

16. A 93-year-old woman is transferred from a nursing home to the emergency room. She is noted to have a core body temperature of 102°F, taken by a rectal thermometer. She is lethargic with a blood pressure of 65/40 mm Hg. A straight catheterization demonstrates increased white blood cells and numerous gram-negative rods. Preliminary blood cultures demonstrate gram-negative rods as well. Which of the following microbial products have likely contributed to her current condition?

    A. Toxic shock syndrome toxin
    B. Lipopolysaccharide (LPS)
    C. Lethal factor
    D. M antigen
    E. Lecithinase

17. A 20-year-old homosexual man presents to the public clinic with a maculopapular rash on his hands and feet. He notes that several weeks ago he had unprotected intercourse with an unknown male at a rave party. A week or two afterward he noted an ulcerative lesion on his penis. He is found to have a positive VDRL test on today's exam. Which of the following is a pathopneumonic lesion in secondary syphilis?

    A. Condyloma acuminata
    B. Gumma
    C. Chancre
    D. Condyloma lata
    E. Tabes dorsalis

18. A 48-year-old AIDS patient presents to the county hospital with complaints of fevers, chills, and night sweats as well as blood-tinged sputum. A chest x-ray demonstrates multiple fine nodules. A CT scan demonstrates fine nodules in the lungs, liver, and bone marrow. His tuberculin test is negative; however, his sputum displays acid-fast bacilli. Which of the following best describes his condition?

    A. Pott disease
    B. Miliary tuberculosis
    C. Primary tuberculosis
    D. Relapsing fever
    E. Scrofula

19. A 25-year-old man returns from a weekend on Cape Cod. He now has colicky abdominal pain and watery diarrhea. He visited a roadside oyster shack with several of his college buddies and all report similar symptoms. In the emergency room, a hepatitis A serology test is negative. He is asked to give a stool sample for culture, which may demonstrate which of the following organisms?

A. *Campylobacter jejuni*
B. *Shigella dysenteriae*
C. *Staphylococcus aureus*
D. *Vibrio parahaemolyticus*
E. *Salmonella typhimurium*

20. A 4-year-old boy is brought to the pediatrician with a runny nose, low-grade fever, myalgias, and headache. He also has a distinctive high-pitched inspiratory whistle with severe paroxysmal coughing fits. He has numerous conjunctival hemorrhages due to his severe cough. Further history reveals he has missed several of his vaccinations. The pediatrician is concerned for whooping cough and prepares a sputum culture. Which is the appropriate medium for the laboratory to culture the sample on?

A. Chocolate agar
B. Cysteine-containing media
C. Thayer–Martin media
D. Bordet–Gengou media
E. MacConkey agar

answers

1-E

A. *Mycobacterium scrofulaceum* [incorrect] is the major cause of scrofula in children. Indeed, it can present with adenopathy of the head and neck. The organism is an acid-fast organism; however, it does not produce "sulfur granules."

B. More commonly seen among immunocompromised patients is *Nocardia asteroides* [incorrect]. This is an anaerobe that is a weakly acid-fast organism that most often causes pneumonia in such patients.

C. Ludwig angina is a potentially life-threatening infection of the mouth that causes swelling of the neck and lower jaw with difficulty swallowing and stridor. It is due to a mixed infection with organisms such as *Bacteroides, Fusobacterium, Treponema* [incorrect], and other oral flora.

D. *Mycobacterium marinum* [incorrect] is a tuberculoid bacterium that causes swimming pool granulomas. These lesions are localized skin infections that develop into purplish nodules that may break down, causing open sores.

E. *Actinomyces israelii* [correct] is an aerobic filamentous branching bacterium that causes cervicofacial, thoracic, abdominal, and pelvic infections. The "sulfur granules" that are associated with infection are really the organism wrapped in calcium phosphate that imparts a yellow sulfur color to the discharge.

2-A

A. The leading cause of endocarditis in intravenous drug users is *Staphylococcus aureus* [correct]. This organism causes acute bacterial endocarditis, affecting even undamaged heart valves. The tricuspid valve is often involved in cases with intravenous drug abusers.

B. *Staphylococcus epidermidis* [incorrect] is a cause of bacterial endocarditis; however, it is typically seen in patients with prosthetic heart valves.

C. Although subacute bacterial endocarditis is most often due to *Streptococcus viridans* [incorrect], in order for vegetations of *S. viridans* to grow, the affected valve must already be damaged.

    D. *Staphylococcus saprophyticus* [incorrect] is a common cause of urinary tract infections.

    E. Although *Streptococcus pneumoniae* [incorrect] does survive in the bloodstream, it is more likely to cause meningitis than endocarditis.

3-E

    A. *Trichomonas vaginalis* [incorrect] is a common sexually transmitted disease that is typified by a watery discharge and the presence of a strawberry cervix. It is a flagellated protozoa that can be seen moving on a wet mount preparation.

    B. The most common sexually transmitted disease is due to *Chlamydia trachomatis* [incorrect]. Infection by these obligate intracellular bacteria can lead to pelvic inflammatory disease with the development of tubo-ovarian abscess, leading to sterility or predisposing one to an ectopic pregnancy.

    C. Pelvic disease due to *Actinomyces israelii* [incorrect] is most often associated with the use of intrauterine devices. A characteristic yellow discharge is common due to sulfur granules.

    D. A common cause of vulvovaginitis is *Candida albicans* [incorrect]. Infection is associated with broad-spectrum antibiotic use, immunocompromised state, and diabetes. The infection results in a cottage-cheese–like discharge, erythema, and pruritus.

    E. A clue cell is a normal vaginal epithelial cell covered with the bacteria, *Gardnerella vaginalis* [correct]. *G. vaginalis* is one of the organisms that contribute to the development of bacterial vaginosis.

4-B

    A. The toxin produced by *Clostridium tetani* [incorrect], tetanus toxin, blocks the release of inhibitory neurotransmitters GABA and glycine at the spinal synapse. This results in a spastic paralysis with rigid muscle contractions.

    B. The toxin produced by *Clostridium botulinum*, botulinum toxin [correct], blocks the release of acetylcholine from the presynaptic neuron, resulting in spastic paralysis. It is associated with infected wounds as well as the ingestion and germination of spores.

    C. Diphtheria toxin [incorrect] is a typical AB toxin produced as a result of a bacteria phage-encoded protein in infected strains of *Corynebacterium diphtheriae*. This toxin blocks protein synthesis by ADP-ribosylation of eukaryotic elongation factor-2 (EF-2).

D. Pertussis toxin [incorrect] is a heat-labile exotoxin that inhibits the actions of an inhibitory G protein, thus resulting in an increase of cyclic AMP (cAMP). Infection by *Bordetella pertussis* results in whopping cough.

E. Cord factor [incorrect] is a virulence factor produced by *Mycobacterium tuberculosis*.

5-A

A. One of the potential complications of *Neisseria gonorrhoeae* [correct] infection is the development of Fitz-Hugh Curtis syndrome. This condition results in acute perihepatitis with "violin string" adhesions.

B. *Ehrlichia chaffeensis* [incorrect] is a gram-negative obligatory intracellular bacteria transmitted by the bite of a tick. It causes human ehrlichiosis characterized by symptoms similar to those of Rocky Mountain spotted fever.

C. Although not a sexually transmitted disease, *Mycobacterium tuberculosis* [incorrect] can cause serious disease in the pelvis, "frozen pelvis." It can cause adhesions within the uterus and fallopian tubes, as well as granulomatous inflammation of the peritoneal lining.

D. Granuloma inguinale [incorrect] is a slowly progressive ulcerative disease involving the genitalia. It is a sexually transmitted disease caused by a gram-negative bacillus, *Calymmatobacterium granulomatis*.

E. *Streptobacillus moniliformis* [incorrect] is the most common cause of rat bite fever in the United States. As well, it causes Haverhill fever and is associated with the consumption of contaminated milk products.

6-D

A. *Bartonella henselae* [incorrect] is a gram-negative rod that causes cat scratch disease as well as bacillary angiomatosis. Cat scratch disease is a cause of lymphadenopathy, particularly in children. Bacillary angiomatosis is a pustular disorder occurring in patients who are immunocompromised (i.e., AIDS patients).

B. Common among rabbit hunters and those who process rabbit pelts, tularemia is caused by the zoonotic organism *Francisella tularensis* [incorrect]. Infection can cause an ulcerative lesion at the site of the skin abrasion, as well as causing influenzalike symptoms with protracted malaise and low-grade fever.

C. Orf [incorrect] is a poxvirus that can cause local ulcerative disease. It is caused by a variola virus that normally infects sheep and goats, so it is more prevalent in ranchers and farmers.

D. The cause of seal finger, or erysipeloid, is the gram-positive bacilli *Erysipelothrix rhusiopathiae* [correct]. It is a common cause of a localized cellulitic infections in fish handlers and meat packers.

E. A zoonotic infection associated with cattle, as well as more recently with bioterrorism, is *Bacillus anthracis* [incorrect], a spore-forming aerobic organism. It can cause cutaneous ulcerative disease as well as severe respiratory infection and gastrointestinal disease.

7-D

A. The toxin produced by *Clostridium tetani* blocks the release of glycine [incorrect]. Glycine is an important inhibitory transmitter at the spinal synapse. Tetanospasmin (tetanus toxin) blocks its release, resulting in spastic paralysis.

B. The toxin produced by *Clostridium botulinum* contains two subunits, the first of which mediates the binding to the cell, and the other blocks the release of acetylcholine [incorrect]. Botulinum toxin causes a flaccid paralysis that can be used therapeutically in the treatment of spastic disorders.

C. *Clostridium perfringens* can cause a serious cellulitis and myonecrosis and is often associated with trauma. This spore-forming organism can germinate in tissue producing a lecithinase, which degrades the surrounding tissue [incorrect].

D. Cholera toxin is a typical AB toxin. The toxin binds to cells and enters. Once inside the toxin, ADP ribosylates the G protein stimulatory protein (Gs), resulting in persistent stimulation signaled by cAMP [correct]. This results in a copious, watery, secretory diarrhea.

E. The toxin produced by *Corynebacterium diphtheriae* can inactivate protein synthesis [incorrect]. It results in the destruction of infected tissue with the formation of pseudomembranes on the throat and tonsils.

8-D

A. Enteropathogenic strains of *Escherichia coli* [incorrect] are often the cause of epidemic infantile diarrhea and nosocomial diarrhea. It destroys the colonic mucosa with resultant watery diarrhea.

B. The most common organism in the human colon is *Bacteroides fragilis* [incorrect]. The obligate anaerobe is a common cause of serious intra-abdominal infection and is often associated with gastrointestinal tract surgery.

C. The most common cause of "traveler's diarrhea" is enterotoxeginic *E. coli* [incorrect]. It produces a toxin similar to cholera toxin, a heat labile toxin that causes a persistent explosive diarrhea with cramping for 1 to 3 days.

D. The boy's presentation is most consistent with infection with an enterohemorrhagic strain of *E. coli* [correct], *E. coli* O157:H7. This strain produces a cytotoxin similar to that of one produced by *Shigella*, resulting in bloody diarrhea. This colitis resolves with the potential appearance of the hemolytic uremic syndrome, characterized by acute renal failure, microangiopathic anemia, and thrombocytopenia.

E. Enteroinvasive strains of *E. coli* [incorrect] are a common cause of dysentery in developing nations.

9-D

A. *Staphylococcus aureus* can cause serious pneumonia and sepsis as well as brain abscesses. The Gram stain of this organism would appear with gram-positive cocci in clusters [incorrect].

B. Gram-positive rods [incorrect] of medical importance include *Bacillus* and *Clostridium*. Although they can cause serious infections, rarely are they the cause of neonatal sepsis or meningitis.

C. Both *Neisseria* and *Haemophilus* are medically important gram-negative cocci [incorrect]. They are important infections with respect to meningitis and respiratory infections. *Neisseria gonorrhoeae* is an important cause of ophthalmia neonatorum, against which all babies born in the United States receive prophylaxis.

D. All of the streptococci stain as gram-positive cocci in chains [correct]. *Streptococcus agalactiae* or group B *Streptococcus* is an important cause of serious neonatal infections. Pregnant women are screened to ascertain if they are carriers of this organism, and if so are given antibiotics prior to delivery.

E. There are numerous medically important gram-negative rods [incorrect], namely the gastrointestinal flora. Indeed, *Escherichia coli* is an important cause of neonatal sepsis and must be considered in such presentations.

10-B

A. Both Arroyo fever and verruga peruana are infections more commonly seen in South America, and are caused by *Bartonella bacilliformis* [incorrect]. This organism is transmitted by the sandfly, the same organism that transmits the protozoal parasite Leishmania.

B. Lyme disease is caused by infection by the spirochete *Borrelia burgdorferi* [correct]. This organism is transmitted by the *Ixodes* tick and is often seen during the summer months, particularly in the northeastern United States.

C. *Ehrlichia chaffeensis* [incorrect] is the cause of human monocytic ehrlichiosis. It is also transmitted by the bite of the *Ixodes* tick, as is the protozoal organism *Babesia microti*.

D. Relapsing fever is a chronic febrile disorder caused by the spirochete *Borrelia recurrentis* [incorrect]. This disease is associated with unsanitary conditions and is transmitted by the bite of a louse.

E. Although *Borrelia burgdorferi* is the cause of Lyme disease, the *Dermacentor* tick [incorrect] is the vector for *Rickettsia rickettsii*, the causative agent of Rocky Mountain spotted fever, and also carries the virus that causes Colorado tick fever.

11-E

A. Rat bite fever is a febrile illness that results from the bite of a rat and infection with *Spirillum minus* [incorrect]. It is more common among laboratory workers, who develop painful rashes in the area of the bite along with tender lymphadenopathy and endocarditis.

B. *Nocardia asteroides* [incorrect] is rarely a cause of infection in immunocompetent individuals. However, in immunocompromised patients, this weakly acid-fast organism can cause fever, pneumonia, and disseminated illness.

C. Often associated with the consumption of contaminated milk and cheese, *Listeria monocytogenes* [incorrect] can cause life-threatening neonatal infections via transplacental transmission. It can also cause pneumonia, conjunctivitis, meningitis, and endocarditis.

D. A component of the flora of human oral cavities, *Streptococcus mutans* [incorrect] is often associated with the development of dental carries.

E. Found in the oral cavity of felines, *Pasteurella multocida* [correct] is often associated with cat bites. As the cat's incisors can penetrate the periosteum of the bone, surgical débridement is required to prevent osteomyelitis.

12-E

A. At one time, *Haemophilus influenzae* [incorrect] was the most common cause of otitis media. However, with the introduction of the preventive vaccine, it is now a rare cause of such infections.

B. *Mycoplasma pneumoniae* [incorrect] is one of the smallest of the free-living bacteria. It is a common cause of community-acquired pneumonia among young adults.

C. *Moraxella catarrhalis* [incorrect] is an organism closely related to *Haemophilus influenzae*. It is a significant cause of otitis media.

D. *Staphylococcus saprophyticus* [incorrect] is a part of the normal skin flora. Unlike *Staphylococcus aureus*, it lacks protein A and coagulase. It is a major cause of urinary tract infections in sexually active females.

E. The leading cause of otitis externa is *Pseudomonas aeruginosa* [correct]. It is often associated with excess moisture in the ear canal and is sometimes known as "swimmer's ear."

13-B

A. The Weil–Felix test [incorrect] is used to detect some rickettsial infections. Infected patients actually produce antibodies that cross-react with the Ox-19 strain of *Proteus*.

B. *Helicobacter pylori* secretes urease and protease, which can break down the gastric mucosa, initiating the development of gastritis. Patients can be given the urease breath test [correct], in which ^{13}C-labelled urea is given, and if *H. pylori* is present, the ^{13}C-labelled urea is broken down to ^{13}C-labeled CO_2 that can be measured in the breath.

C. The Whiff test [incorrect] is performed by adding several drops of KOH to a wet mount of vaginal secretions. The production of a fishy odor indicates the presence of bacterial vaginosis.

D. The Mantoux test [incorrect] is performed by injecting a small amount of tuberculin or purified protein derivative (PPD) subcutaneously. If patients have been exposed to tuberculosis, they will develop a delayed-type hypersensitivity reaction indicated by induration at the injection site.

E. Used to detect the presence of lecithinase, the Nagler reaction [incorrect] aids in the confirmation of *Clostridium perfringens* infection.

14-C

A. Gram-negative kidney-shaped diplococci [incorrect] can be found both extracellularly and within neutrophils in the purulent urethral discharge of *Neisseria gonorrhoeae* infections.

B. *Clostridium tetani* appears as gram-positive rods with terminal spores [incorrect], that often resemble tennis rackets.

C. One of the leading causes of pneumonia is *Streptococci pneumoniae*. These organisms can be detected in Gram stains of sputum cultures as gram-positive lancet-shaped diplococci [correct].

D. Often associated with contaminated drinking water, *Vibrio cholerae* is a major cause of diarrhea worldwide. These organisms appear as gram-negative comma-shaped organisms [incorrect].

E. A common cause of aspiration pneumonia in alcoholics is the enteric bacterium *Klebsiella pneumoniae*. This organism is a gram-negative rod with a thick mucoid capsule [incorrect].

15-D

A. Scalded skin syndrome [incorrect] is an exfoliative dermatitis that spreads over the body as a sunburn-type rash. It is due to the elaboration of an exotoxin by *Staphylococcus aureus*.

B. An acute inflammatory reaction of the superficial layers of the skin, erysipelas [incorrect] manifests with a plaquelike rash. It is usually associated with group A *Streptococcus* infection.

C. Toxic shock syndrome [incorrect] is associated with a high fever, vomiting, and diarrhea. It results from the production of a superantigen by *S. aureus*, and is more commonly seen in menstruating women in association with tampon or contraceptive sponge use.

D. Impetigo [correct] is a self-limited illness associated with streptococci. The same strain of *Streptococcus* is associated with the development of post-streptococcal glomerulonephritis.

E. Scarlet fever [incorrect] results in an extensive erythematous rash as well as the presence of a "strawberry tongue." Due to group A β-hemolytic *Streptococcus pyogenes*, these patients would have elevated ASO titers.

16-B

A. Toxic shock syndrome toxin (TSST) [incorrect] is produced by *Staphylococcus aureus* and functions as a superantigen. As such, it is a polyclonal activator of T cells, resulting in a fever and a rash.

B. Present in the cell wall of gram-negative bacteria, lipopolysaccharide (LPS) [correct] triggers the release of tumor necrosis factor and interleukin-1 from immune system cells. This leads to life-threatening distributive shock.

C. Part of the trivalent anthrax toxin, lethal factor [incorrect] causes the CNS depression seen with *Bacillus anthracis* infection. The other two toxins produced by anthrax are protective antigen and edema factor.

D. Found in the cell wall of *Streptococcus pyogenes*, M antigen [incorrect] is an important virulence factor. It is thought that rheumatic heart disease results from antibodies against M antigen that cross-react with heart valve tissue, resulting in damage to heart valves.

E. An important virulence factor for *Clostridium perfringens* is lecithinase [incorrect]. This enzyme degrades tissue and is associated with myonecrosis.

17-D

A. Condyloma acuminatum [incorrect] is a warty cauliflowerlike lesion that develops as a result of human papillomavirus (HPV) infection.

B. A gumma [incorrect] is a white-gray rubbery tumorlike mass that can develop in the liver, skin, or bones. It is the result of granulomatous inflammation associated with tertiary syphilis.

C. Two to ten weeks following infection with *Treponema pallidum,* an ulcerative lesion can form. This lesion, known as a chancre [incorrect], is the typical lesion of primary syphilis.

D. Along with the maculopapular rash, secondary syphilis presents with condyloma lata [correct]. This lesion is a gray, flattened wartlike lesion in the anogenital, axillary, or oral region.

E. Tabes dorsalis [incorrect] results as part of the sequelae of a syphilis infection. It manifests with reduced positional and vibrational sense in the lower extremities, as well as loss of deep tendon reflexes. It is present in tertiary syphilis and results from demyelination and axonal loss in the dorsal roots and columns.

18-B

A. When tuberculosis infects the vertebrae it is known as Pott disease [incorrect]. This condition results in extensive involvement of the medullary cavity with the development of compression fractures and contiguous spread to the psoas muscle with abscess formation.

B. Once tuberculosis reactivates, it can go on to hematogenously spread to other organs throughout the body. With miliary tuberculosis [correct], organs like the spleen, liver, and bone marrow become involved in a grossly visible caseating necrosis that presents with the appearance of millet seeds on gross inspection of the involved organs.

C. Primary infection with tuberculosis [incorrect] usually results in a localized parenchymal scar, as well as calcified lymph nodes, the so-called Ghon complex.

D. Relapsing fever [incorrect] is a louse-borne disease caused by *Borrelia recurrentis*. It is characterized by high fever, shaking chills, headache, and diarrhea.

E. A related organism to *Mycobacterium tuberculosis* is *M. scrofulaceum* [incorrect]. In children, the condition results in painless cervical adenopathy, which can ulcerate with sinus tract formation.

19-D

A. A common cause of bloody diarrhea is *Campylobacter jejuni* [incorrect]. As the organism invades the mucosa, a smear of the stool will demonstrate leukocytes along with gull wing–shaped gram-negative bacilli.

B. *Shigella dysenteriae* [incorrect] is associated with a low-volume bloody diarrhea. It produces a toxin, Shiga toxin, which can inactivate protein synthesis.

C. *Staphylococcus aureus* [incorrect] can cause vomiting, cramps, and diarrhea. It is often the result of preformed toxin on meats, dairy products, salad dressings, and cream salads, but manifests within 2 to 8 hours of consumption.

D. The halophilic organism *Vibrio parahaemolyticus* [correct] is often associated with seafood consumption. A watery diarrhea results from the production of an enterotoxin.

E. Commonly associated with the consumption of eggs, poultry, and meat, *Salmonella typhimurium* [incorrect] can cause a bloody diarrhea. Patients with low gastric acidity (e.g., pernicious anemia) are at a greater risk of infection.

20-D

A. *Haemophilus influenzae* used to be a major cause of many childhood infections, including otitis media and epiglottitis, until the introduction of the preventive vaccine. It, however, remains a significant pathogen in older patients with lung disease, and its isolation is performed on chocolate agar [incorrect] that provides the factor V and X required for bacterial growth.

B. *Legionella pneumoniae* is another important cause of pneumonia in older patients, and is partially associated with standing water in cooling towers or air conditioning systems. It requires cysteine [incorrect] for growth.

C. *Neisseria* species, both meningococcal and gonococcal, are selected by growth on Thayer–Martin media [incorrect].

D. The cause of whooping cough as presented in the vignette is *Bordetella pertussis*. This gram-negative cocci grows best on Bordet–Gengou media [correct].

E. MacConkey agar [incorrect] is a general purpose media for growth of gram-negative bacteria. It contains a dye that changes to red when the organism can ferment lactose (e.g., *Escherichia coli* and *Klebsiella*), and remains white when the organism cannot ferment lactose (as is the case with *Salmonella* and *Shigella*).

credits

Armitage JO, Antman KH. *High-Dose Cancer Therapy: Pharmacology, Hematopoietins, Stem Cells, 3rd ed.* Philadelphia: Lippincott Williams & Wilkins, 2000. Fig. 16 – Ch 35 (Case 32).

Avner ED, Harmon WE, Niaudet P. *Pediatric Nephrology, 5th ed.* Philadelphia: Lippincott Williams & Wilkins, 2003. Figs. 47.4 (Case 35), 24.18 (Case 66).

Bailey BJ, Johnson JT, et al. *Head and Neck Surgery—Otolaryngology, 4th ed.* Philadelphia: Lippincott Williams & Wilkins, 2006. Fig. 135.5 (Case 56).

Becker KL, Bilezikian JP, Brenner WJ, et al. *Principles and Practice of Endocrinology and Metabolism, 3rd ed.* Philadelphia: Lippincott Williams & Wilkins, 2001. Fig. 83-2 (Case 48).

Betts RF, Chapman SW, Penn RL. *Reese & Betts': A Practical Approach to Infectious Disease, 5th ed.* Philadelphia: Lippincott Williams & Wilkins, 2001:T13.4 (Case 96).

Bhushan V, Le T, Pall V. *Underground Clinical Vignettes: Step One—Microbiology II, 4th ed.* Malden, Mass: Blackwell Publishing, 2005. Figs. 011 (Case 11), 036 A & B (Case 31), 046 A & B (Case 40), 048 (Case 42), 097 (Case 84), 100 (Case 88).

Centers for Disease Control and Prevention: Public Health Image Library (PHIL). Figs. 6654.tif (Case 17), 6378.jpeg (Case 98).

Cohen WR. *Cherry and Merkatz's Complications of Pregnancy, 5th ed.* Philadelphia: Lippincott Williams & Wilkins, 1999. Fig. 34-19 (Case 30).

DeLisa JA, Gans BM, et al. *Physical Medicine and Rehabilitation: Principles and Practice, 4th ed.* Philadelphia: Lippincott Williams & Wilkins, 2004. Fig. 33-6B (Case 19).

Eisenberg RL. *Clinical Imaging: An Atlas of Differential Diagnosis, 4th ed.* Philadelphia: Lippincott Williams & Wilkins, 2002. Figs. C 9-1B (Case 8), SK 6-10B (Case 14), C 44-8 (Case 90).

Elder DE, Elenitsas R, et al. *Lever's Histopathology of the Skin, 9th ed.* Philadelphia: Lippincott Williams & Wilkins, 2004. Figs. 21-22 (Case 9), 21-13 (Case 91).

Engleberg NC, Dermody T, DiRita V. *Schaechter's Mechanisms of Microbial Disease, 4th ed.* Philadelphia: Lippincott Williams & Wilkins, 2006. Figs. 57-7 (Case 13), 22-1 (Case 38), 29-1 (Case 49), 24-2 (Case 85), T63-1 (Case 94), T63-2 (Case 95).

Fisher RG, Boyce TG. *Moffet's Pediatric Infectious Diseases: A Problem-Oriented Approach, 4th ed.* Philadelphia: Lippincott Williams & Wilkins, 2004. Figs. 2-8 (Case 22), 11-1 (Case 77).

Fleisher GR, Ludwig S, Baskin MN. *Atlas of Pediatric Emergency Medicine.* Philadelphia: Lippincott Williams & Wilkins, 2004. Figs. 11:19B (Case 24), 11:47 (Case 75).

Fleisher GR, Ludwig S, Baskin MN. *Textbook of Pediatric Emergency Medicine.* Philadelphia: Lippincott Williams & Wilkins, 2004. Figs. 101.16 (Case 44), 84.7 (Case 57), 84.6 (Case 63), 94.13 A & B (Case 85).

Gorbach SL, Bartlett JG, Blacklow NR. *Infectious Diseases, 3rd ed.* Philadelphia: Lippincott Williams & Wilkins, 2003. Figs. 221.3 (Case 1), 73.4 (Case 20), 183.4 (Case 25), 158.12 (Case 39), 167.1 (Case 73), 164.2 (Case 92).

Greenberg MJ, Hendrickson RG. *Greenberg's Text-Atlas of Emergency Medicine.* Philadelphia: Lippincott Williams & Wilkins, 2004. Figs. 20-17B (Case 7), 20-18 (Case 18), 1-5A (Case 24), 26-11 (Case 26).

Greenspan A. *Orthopedic Imaging: A Practical Approach, 4th ed.* Philadelphia: Lippincott Williams & Wilkins, 2004. Fig. 25.2B (Case 55).

Hall JC. *Sauer's Manual of Skin Disorders, 9th ed.* Philadelphia: Lippincott Williams & Wilkins, 2006. Fig. 38-1 (Case 12).

Hickey JV. *Clinical Practice of Neurological and Neurosurgical Nursing, 5th ed.* Philadelphia: Lippincott Williams & Wilkins, 2002. Figs. 30-1 (Case 45), 30-2 (Case 47).

Humes HD. *Kelley's Textbook of Internal Medicine, 2nd ed.* Philadelphia: Lippincott Williams & Wilkins, 2001. Figs. 288.2 (Case 33), 297.3 (Case 37), 275.3 (Case 51), 301.1 (Case 53), 270.1 (Case 69), 298.1 (Case 99).

Irwin RS, Cerra FB, Rippe JM. *Irwin & Rippe's Intensive Care Medicine, 5th ed.* Philadelphia: Lippincott Williams & Wilkins, 2003. Figs. 67-12 (Case 6), 81-1 (Case 81).

Keyes DC, Burstein JL, et al. *Medical Response to Terrorism: Preparedness and Clinical Practice.* Philadelphia: Lippincott Williams & Wilkins, 2004. Fig. 7-5 (Case 64).

Koopman WJ, Moreland LW. *Arthritis and Allied Conditions: A Textbook of Rheumatology, 15th ed.* Philadelphia: Lippincott Williams & Wilkins, 2004. Fig. 64.1 (Case 100).

Lee JK, Sagel SS, et al. *Computed Body Tomography with MRI Correlation, 4th ed.* Philadelphia: Lippincott Williams & Wilkins, 2005. Figs. 11-77 (Case 52), 24-77 (Case 70), 16-26 (Case 82).

Loeser JD. *Bonica's Management of Pain, 3rd ed.* Philadelphia: Lippincott Williams & Wilkins, 2000:T66-1 (Case 62).

McMillan JA, Fergin RD, et al. *Oski's Pediatrics: Principles and Practice, 4th ed.* Philadelphia: Lippincott Williams & Wilkins, 2006. Figs. 229.1 (Case 3), 68.13 (Case 36), 116.7 (Case 43), 156.1 (Case 44), T61-6.8 (Case 45), T172.1 (Case 72), 68.13 (Case 76), 81.3 (Case 83), 81.5 (Case 83-2).

Menkes JH, Sarnat HB, Maria BL. *Child Neurology, 7th ed.* Philadelphia: Lippincott Williams & Wilkins, 2005. Fig. 10.3 (Case 87).

Oldham KT, Colombani PM, et al. *Principles and Practice of Pediatric Surgery.* Philadelphia: Lippincott Williams & Wilkins, 2004. Fig. 79-3 (Case 50).

Rock JA, Jones III HW. *Te Linde's Operative Gynecology, 9th ed.* Philadelphia: Lippincott Williams & Wilkins, 2003. Fig. 28.11 (Case 61).

Rowland LP. *Merritt's Neurology, 11th ed.* Philadelphia: Lippincott Williams & Wilkins, 2005. Fig. 28.1 A (Case 86).

Rubin E, Gorstein F, Schwarting R, et al. *Rubin's Pathology: A Clinicopathologic Approach, 4th ed.* Baltimore: Lippincott Williams & Wilkins, 2004. Figs. 11-36 (Case 2), 11-30 (Case 5), 9-24 (Case 20), 18-2 (Case 60), 7-34 (Case 79), 9-28 (Case 88), 9-47 (Case 90).

Schiff ER, Sorrell MF, Maddrey WC. *Schiff's Diseases of the Liver, 9th ed.* Philadelphia: Lippincott Williams & Wilkins, 2003. Figs. 59.3 (Case 16), 8B.38 (Case 71).

Singleton JK, Sandowski SA, et al. *Primary Care.* Philadelphia: Lippincott Williams & Wilkins, 1999. Fig. 68-1 (Case 68).

Sweet RL, Gibbs RS. *Infectious Diseases of the Female Genital Tract, 4th ed.* Philadelphia: Lippincott Williams & Wilkins, 2001. Figs. 20.9 (Case 17), 5.5 (Case 27).

Wachter RM, Goldman L, Hollander H. *Hospital Medicine, 2nd ed.* Philadelphia: Lippincott Williams & Wilkins, 2005. Fig. 77.5, T77.5 (Case 17).

Wolfson AB, Hendey GW, et al. *Harwood-Nuss' Clinical Practice of Emergency Medicine, 4th ed.* Philadelphia: Lippincott Williams & Wilkins, 2005. Figs. 261.1 (Case 65), 126.3 A & B (Case 89).

Yamada T, Alpers DH, et al. *Textbook of Gastroenterology, 4th ed.* Philadelphia: Lippincott Williams & Wilkins, 2003. Figs. 68-3 (Case 62), 142-52 (Case 74).

case list

BACTERIOLOGY

1. Actinomycosis
2. Acute Bacterial Endocarditis
3. Acute Bronchiolitis
4. Acute Cystitis
5. Acute Rheumatic Fever
6. Acute Sinusitis
7. Anthrax
8. Aspiration Pneumonia with Abscess
9. Atypical Mycobacterial Infection
10. *Bacillus cereus* Food Poisoning
11. Bacterial Vaginosis
12. Bartonellosis
13. Botulism
14. Brain Abscess
15. Breast Abscess
16. Brucellosis
17. Campylobacter Enteritis
18. Cat-Scratch Disease
19. Cellulitis
20. Cholera
21. Chorioamnionitis
22. Diphtheria
23. Ehrlichiosis
24. Epiglottitis
25. Erysipelas
26. Erysipeloid
27. Fitz–Hugh–Curtis Syndrome
28. Gas Gangrene—Traumatic
29. Gastroenteritis—*Staphylococcus aureus*
30. Gonococcal Ophthalmia Neonatorum
31. Gonorrhea
32. Graft-Versus-Host Disease
33. Granuloma Inguinale
34. *Haemophilus influenzae* Infection in a COPD Patient
35. Hemolytic-Uremic Syndrome (HUS)
36. Impetigo
37. Jarisch-Herxheimer Reaction
38. *Legionella* Pneumonia
39. Leprosy—Lepromatous
40. Leprosy—Tuberculoid
41. Leptospirosis (Weil Disease)
42. *Listeria* Meningitis in the Newborn
43. Listeriosis
44. Lyme Disease
45. Meningitis—Bacterial (Adult)
46. Meningitis—Bacterial (Pediatric)
47. Meningitis—Tubercular
48. Meningococcemia
49. Mycoplasma Pneumonia
50. Necrotizing Enterocolitis
51. Necrotizing Fasciitis
52. Neutropenic Enterocolitis
53. Nocardiosis
54. Nosocomial Enterococcal Infection
55. Osteomyelitis
56. Otitis Externa
57. Otitis Media
58. Overwhelming Postsplenectomy Infection
59. *Pasteurella multocida*
60. Pelvic Inflammatory Disease
61. Pelvic Tuberculosis
62. Peptic Ulcer Disease (*Helicobacter pylori*)
63. Pharyngitis—Streptococcal
64. Plague

65. Pneumococcal Pneumonia
66. Poststreptococcal Glomerulonephritis
67. Prostatitis—Acute
68. Prostatitis—Chronic
69. Prosthetic Valve Endocarditis
70. Pyelonephritis—Acute
71. Pyogenic Liver Abscess
72. Rat Bite Fever
73. Relapsing Fever
74. *Salmonella* Food Poisoning
75. *Salmonella* Septicemia with Osteomyelitis
76. Scalded Skin Syndrome
77. Scarlet Fever
78. Shigellosis
79. Shock—Septic
80. Spontaneous Bacterial Peritonitis
81. Subacute Bacterial Endocarditis
82. Subdiaphragmatic Abscess
83. Syphilis—Congenital
84. Syphilis—Primary
85. Syphilis—Secondary
86. Syphilis—Tertiary
87. Tetanus
88. Tetanus Neonatorum
89. Toxic Shock Syndrome (TSS)
90. Tuberculosis—Miliary
91. Tuberculosis—Pulmonary
92. Tularemia
93. Typhoid Fever
94. Urinary Tract Infection (UTI)
95. UTI with *Staphylococcus saprophyticus*
96. *Vibrio parahaemolyticus* Food Poisoning
97. *Vibrio vulnificus* Food Poisoning
98. Whooping Cough
99. Yaws
100. Yersinia Enterocolitis

index